Between Dancing and Writing

Between Dancing and Writing

THE PRACTICE OF RELIGIOUS STUDIES

Kimerer L. LaMothe

FORDHAM UNIVERSITY PRESS   NEW YORK   2004

Library of Congress Cataloging-in-Publication Data

LaMothe, Kimerer L.
    Between dancing and writing: the practice of
religious studies / Kimerer L. LaMothe.— 1st ed.
        p. cm.
    Includes bibliographical references and index.
    ISBN 0-8232-2403-1 (hardcover)
    1. Religion—Philosophy. 2. Dance—Religious aspects.
3. Religious dance, Modern. I. Title.
    BL51.L365 2004
    200'.7—dc22

Printed in the United States of America
07 06 05 04 5 4 3 2 1

First edition

Contents

Acknowledgements

Faced with the task of acknowledging the people who have enabled the event of this book, I cannot help thinking about a quotation from Nietzsche's *Ecce Homo*: "How could I fail to be grateful to my whole life?"

This book is, in a sense, about my whole life. It is a living link between communities whose members meet in its pages—teachers, mentors, colleagues, and friends in the worlds of dance and religious studies.

Preliminary movements towards this book began in my work with Mark C. Taylor and H. Gans Little at Williams College. In their classes, I first called upon dance as a resource for addressing post-modern critiques of onto-theology. I am grateful for their ongoing encouragement.

In the course of graduate work, larger written gestures received invaluable support from Gordon Kaufman, Lawrence Sullivan, Margaret Miles, Sharon Welch, John Carman, Francis Fiorenza, Stanley Cavell, and Diane Apostolos-Cappadona.

Along the way, my experience of dance deepened and developed in work with Sharron Rose, Marcus Schulkind, the Martha Graham School of Contemporary Dance and its teachers, especially Maher Benham, Denise Vale, and Pearl Lang.

The manuscript assumed its current shape during my year as a fellow at the Radcliffe Institute for Advanced Study in 2000-2001. I am deeply grateful to Director Rita Nakashima Brock for her visionary support of both my writing and dancing, as well as to the Office for the Arts at Harvard University and its Director of Dance, Elizabeth Bergmann.

Under the auspices of a Fortieth Anniversary Fellowship from the Religion and Arts Initiative of the Center for the Study of World Religions, the manuscript received a final polish. Special thanks to Diana Eck, Alison Edwards, and the Center staff, as well as to my editor at Fordham, Helen Tartar, and the readers whose comments guided the process.

The wisdom of friends and family has enriched the progress of this book every step of the way. I am indebted to Kathleen Skerrett, Colby Devitt, Deborah Abel, Sharron Rose, Miranda Shaw, Alexis McCrossen, Courtney Bickel Lamberth, and R. Marie Griffith. To my parents, Cynthia and Jack LaMothe, for always being there, to John LaMothe for the cover photograph, and to the students and colleagues at Harvard who have challenged my thinking, thank you.

Finally, my life partner Geoff Gee, a musician, was the first person to read the manuscript in its entirety. His belief in the value of my writing and dancing is a "disconcerting miracle" I never fail to appreciate. My children, Jordan, Jessica, and Kyra, remind me constantly how vital it is to do what we can to envision better futures. I dedicate the book to this family who makes everything possible.

Preface
Moving Between

All good things approach their goal crookedly. Like cats, they arch their backs, they purr inwardly over their approaching happiness: all good things laugh.

— Friedrich Nietzsche, *Thus Spoke Zarathustra*[1]

People have asked me why I chose to be a dancer. I did not choose. I was chosen to be a dancer, and with that, you live all your life.

— Martha Graham, *Blood Memory*[2]

At first I tried to choose. I wanted to choose. I thought I had to choose between being a dancer and being a scholar of religion—that is, between the study and practice of modern dance and the study and practice of Christian theology and philosophy of religion. It seemed obvious. As conceived and lived in the modern West, the worlds of dance and religious studies move in opposite directions: artistic versus intellectual; embodied versus mental; feminine versus masculine; outwardly performative versus inwardly transforming. They represent discrete cultures and community networks, different in their styles of dress, codes of behavior, hierarchies of values, and architectural demands. Participation in either discipline requires total commitment.

Educated to believe in the range of conceptual distinctions that justified the separation of these worlds, I was not surprised that I constantly felt torn in my attempt to move between them. In dance class, I could not help thinking about books I should be reading; in the lecture hall, I chafed against the imposed stillness, yearning to move vividly and put ideas into action. To me, this sense of tearing was proof that I had to choose. For years, I yearned for simplicity—to want to do only one thing. I tried to excise the pull of one or the other practice from my life, and just dance or just study religion. At every turn, the effort backfired, impelling me reluctantly and eagerly back to the field whose claims on my time and energy I sought to repress.

Slowly the realization dawned: I could not choose. Each activity attunes me to a dimension of life without which a day is not complete. When I practice dance, whether European or American, Haitian or Hindu, sensory capacities breathe into awareness, opening onto new shapes of strength and kinetic potential. Releasing into the movement invites a rush of energy, a sense of body flowing, touching, becoming life. When reading theologians and philosophers of religion I am dazzled with ways of imagining the world that alter my sense of what is possible and desirable, meaningful and true. Many texts have guided me towards unforeseen horizons of understanding. Each activity then honors a capacity for experience and expression; each stirs and engages dimensions of consciousness that cooperate in the project of making and valuing life. How could I choose? The pull I have felt between dancing and writing comprises a *generative paradox* at the heart of my life, an irreducible tension held together by the passion of necessity. Following Nietzsche's advice, I have learned to laugh at my crooked path.

■ ■ ■

This book represents an early fruit of my efforts to live this generative paradox. It recounts my effort to discern why scholars in the field of religious studies tend to devalue "dance," or rhythmic bodily movement, in relation to text-friendly forms of religious life. Even in cases where scholars notice and describe dancing, I find something missing: an account of the contribution that the *action* of dancing makes to the religious meaning of the event at hand. In most cases, dances are described as texts, as functioning like texts, as enacting or imitating texts, or as explained with reference to texts, textual metaphors, or text-based methods of interpretation. Of course, in the tomes of modern Christian theology and philosophy, dance hardly appears at all.

Or does it? The aim of this book is to unsettle the perception that dance is marginal to the practice and thus the study of religions. Along the way I advance a startling thesis: a mutually generative relationship between what appears as "religion" and what appears as "dance" lies at the heart of modern Western theories and methods of religious studies. Not only are our conceptions of the relationship between religion and dance negotiable, but this negotiation is necessary in order to enhance our understanding of religion in its conceptual, bodily, and historical forms. Religious studies scholars, I argue, stand to benefit from attending to dancing as a medium of religious experience and expression: we will find resources in the practices of dance for addressing important debates in the field today concerning the role of bodily being in religious life, and the relation of theory and theology in religious studies.

■ ■ ■

Impelling the argument in this book is my own ongoing movement between the practices of dancing and of reading and writing about religion. Moving between them, I have discovered a process they share. Each activity presents me, indeed calls me into the present, though differently. Each exercises a full spectrum of human sensibilities—kinesthetic, sensory, emotional, and intellectual. Each animates a different sense of self in relation to others and the world. I find myself between writing and dancing.

Moving between these practices has helped me appreciate the impact what we do has on what we think.³ I have come to believe that the idea that religion and dance are mutually exclusive activities itself represents someone's sense of bodily self. It represents a sense of self as a mental activity capable of operating independently of bodily sense and context. It represents a sense of self and world cultivated by those who practice reading and writing as the condition for their success.

Said otherwise, my movement between the practices of dancing and religious studies provides me with a perspective from which to interpret as *significant* the conceptual and institutional gaps in modern western culture between dance and religion. These gaps are not products of a "natural" distinction between mind and body, or between words and gestures. These gaps are a function of our faith in the practice of writing. In practicing writing, we are encouraged to forget that the marginal location of dance in western culture derives from the systems of belief, practice, and education that develop citizens into readers and writers. We are educated to believe that the "truth," even about dance, finds its authority in the medium of verbal language. In such an economy, as some have criticized and others celebrated, dance eludes representation.

However, contrary to common perception, dance does not elude representation because it is "non-verbal" or bodily. To perceive dancing as "nonverbal" is not to see dancing; it is to see (from the perspective of one who uses) verbal language. Dancing appears as a "non," a primitive or derivative form of what can otherwise be represented in words. Correlatively, those who privilege dance because it is nonverbal do so at the expense of their ability to acknowledge dance as a medium of experience and expression in its own right. They have already assumed the perspective of the verbal economy in which dance has no voice.⁴

From the perspective enabled by my movement between practices, by contrast, dancing eludes verbal representation because it exercises different patterns of mental and physical coordination than those required to read and write. Dancing marks the limit of what writing can capture and represent. Yet this limit is not one defined by content—as if dance represented an "object" or symbolic meaning that refuses translation into the medium of words. Dancing marks the limit of writing in so far as it represents an alternative "disciplinary practice" to that represented by reading and writing about religion.[5] Dancing communicates participation in the realm of action and thinking which its practice and performance open within the person who dances. From this perspective, what appears as "dance" and what appears as "religion" draw near indeed. The perception of the gap between them appears as a sign of what they share. Our contemporary experience of each is implicated in the life of writing. This book is an extended mediation on this nexus of ideas.

■ ■ ■

A question arises: if dance eludes verbal representation, how then can I *write* about *dance* in a way that allows it to appear as a medium of knowledge on its own terms? My primary strategy is to continue my own practice of dancing. I keep moving between dancing and writing, keeping the sensibilities required to dance alive in the body that sits and thinks.

Doing so helps me remember. I remember that what appears on the page is mediated by the capacities opened in me by my experiences of dancing, even as my experiences of dancing are informed by my intellectual reflections on what I am doing. I remember that in the process of writing about religion, I produce myself as a dancer, and in my dancing, I render myself capable of writing about religion. I remember how I cannot not try to articulate in writing the impact that my dancing continues to exert on my thinking about religion—and vice versa.

Thus, I write about dance knowing that what I can think and write about "it" does not exhaust the forms in which my knowledge about religion and dance appears, and that what I can think and write does not represent all that can be known about dancing or even necessarily what is most important to know about dancing. I write what I can write. I seek to persuade readers of the generative paradox between dancing and writing that informs this project in religious studies. My hope is that readers will feel compelled to take breaks from their reading and move; that they will embrace the possibility that the practice of attending to their own embodied movement can enrich their scholarly understanding of religious phenomena.

■ ■ ■

Attention to the practice and performance of dance for those working within the study of religion, within the academy, and within the culture at large is crucial. Without the effort to remember dance as something other than nonverbal bodily action, the paradox between dancing and writing which feeds our reading-writing-thinking selves loses degrees of generativity. Persons become increasingly out of touch—even in the attempt to be in touch—with the rhythms of physical living that comprise human vitality. The perception and real manifestation of a mutual distinction between writing and dancing is a cultural conceit with a history for which we must account. While there can be no return to a culture in which writing does not dominate human consciousness, there can be movement forward towards an appreciation and practice of writing as itself a kind of dancing, and of dancing as a medium of religious experience and expression.

Between Dancing and Writing

Introduction
A Disconcerting Miracle

This book sets an agenda for an emerging area of scholarship in the field of religious studies: the philosophy of religion and dance. It provides scholars in the field, whether historians, humanists, social scientists, or theologians, with the theoretical resources they need to recognize why and how a given instance of "dance" is significant for what they perceive as "religion."

Religion and dance? The incredulous responses to such a pairing are by now familiar. Are the two even related? As the reaction is common among scholars and dancers, family and friends, regardless of profession or religious commitment, I marvel at how commonplace it is among citizens of modern western culture to consider "religion" and "dance" as mutually exclusive spheres of human activity. For most people—religious studies scholars included—"dance" conjures up images of bodies moving in space, most often female bodies, sweaty and stretched, on display in ballet and burlesque, in dance clubs and social gatherings, as art and entertainment. Dance appears as the ultimate play, a way to spend leisure time after the work is done. By contrast, "religion" calls to mind beliefs and practices oriented toward ultimate truths. "Religion" addresses spiritual and social concerns; it demands commitment, community, and discipline. In religion, people still their bodies and raise their hearts and minds in devotion. In dance they still their minds and release their bodies. Indeed, what can dance and religion have in common?

Such reactions confirm the importance of this project, for the perception of dance and religion as mutually exclusive activities is an anomaly when seen in the context of world history. Dance—defined here as *rhythmic bodily movement*, whether spontaneous or rehearsed, choreographed or improvised, performed alone, with accompaniment, or among others—is present in some strand of nearly every major world tradition, and most known indigenous cultures. People around the world and throughout time have practiced some kind of *rhythmic bodily movement* as effective for the kinds of experience and expression studied by western scholars under the category of "religion." Even Christian history, contrary to popular impression, is alive with a rich if conflicted legacy of attitudes towards dance. Nowhere, for example, does the Bible forbid or condemn "dance." Various accounts of leaping, jumping, whirling, processing, and gesturing are encouraged and defended.[1] Even in the modern period when scholars concur that Christian authorities effectively purged dance from the mainstreams of Protestant and Catholic practice, dancing continues to pop up in the heat of revivals (such as those in eighteenth- and nineteenth-century United States), in marginalized and millennial sects (such as the early Quakers and the Shakers), or in encultured or syncretic liturgies (such as the "Shout" of African-American Christians, and the dance liturgies in Africa and Indonesia).[2] Given the ubiquity of dancing in religious life, it follows that the ability to understand when, how, why, and to what effect people dance should be crucial to projects in the field of religious studies.[3]

Nevertheless, the field of religious studies took root in a cultural context where the intellectual and religious elites, if they considered "dancing" an art at all, considered it a lesser or derivative art.[4] Early scholars in religious studies, in turn, were so successful in their attempts to reproduce a perception of religion and dance as antithetical that many now understand it to be the normal state of affairs in relation to the two practices. Although scholars of religion may notice dance and may even provide vivid descriptions of actual dancing, the field has not yet developed conceptual tools for articulating the contributions to religious life made by the act of dancing. "Dance" appears as "religion" when it conforms to a given theory of what religion is.

Towards developing a philosophy, or more precisely, a phenomenology of religion and dance, this book undertakes two tasks. The first, occupying Part 1, is to discern reasons why scholars intent on studying "religion" have failed to take adequate account of dance. In this regard I revisit formative moments in the pre-history of the field of religious studies, and identify dynamics internal to the emerging project of using the word "religion" which have served to divert attention from the idea that dance may in fact be religion. In the process I challenge a dominant narrative of the history of the field of religious studies—what I call the "emergence narrative." According to the emergence narrative, *Religionswissenschaft* was conceived by Christian theologians, born in Christian institutions, funded by theological concepts, and guided by theological interests. It establishes itself as a scholarly discipline in so far as it completes its emergence from, over, and against "theology."[5] Adherence to this emergence narrative, I argue, hinders attention to rhythmic bodily movement as a medium of religious experience and expression.

My second task, occupying Part 2, is to document an approach to religious studies in which theology and theory coexist in a generative tension, and to demonstrate how such an approach opens the possibility for considering dance not only as a medium of religious experience and expression, but also as a resource for generating theory and method in the study of religion. In other words, I am interested in how thinking about dance as religion can stretch and reform our understanding of "religion" and not just of "dance." For help in this task I call upon the Dutch phenomenologist, Christian theologian, and historian of religions, Gerardus van der Leeuw (1890–1950). Van der Leeuw developed a braided methodological approach to the study of religion in which his unique phenomenology of religion functions as a mediating thread, weaving between theological projects and historical studies. The value of his approach is evident in the wealth of conceptual resources he generates for thinking about moments in time when something appears to someone as both dance and religion. He calls such a moment, for reasons that will become clear, a "disconcerting miracle."[6]

COMPLICATING THE EMERGENCE NARRATIVE

The reason I devote so much of this book to identifying dynamics internal to the field that enforce a perception of religion and dance as mutually opposing is that contemporary scholars interested in dance and the bodily dimensions of religious life more generally have tended to underestimate how deeply the resistance to considering dance as religion penetrates their field. Correlatively, scholars tend to underestimate the magnitude of the changes in theory and method needed in order to esteem dance. Their subsequent attempts to embrace dance unwittingly reinforce and even justify its marginal status in the life of "religion."

The most familiar and best example of this dynamic occurs among those who invoke an emergence narrative of the field to critique the dearth of attention paid by scholars to the physical, aesthetic, and nontextual aspects of religious life.[7] A number of scholars have argued that a lingering Protestant paradigm causes scholars in the field to favor verbal media and verbal practices over other forms of religious communication. Scholars' theological bias appears in the objects they choose to study (scriptures, doctrine, beliefs); in the methods they bring to bear on these objects (linguistic, structural, or interpretive); in the training prescribed for scholars (learning languages, reading and writing books); and in the desired goals and products of scholarship (books, lectures, and syllabi). In the context of a

Protestant paradigm, rhythmic bodily action can appear only as what Michel Foucault calls a "subjugated knowledge." Not only are historical moments of dancing "buried and disguised," but dance in general is "disqualified" as a "naive knowledge . . . located low down on the hierarchy, beneath the required level of cognition or scientificity."[8] In sum, for those who adhere to the emergence narrative, the kind of attention dance has received in religious studies offers one more proof that the study of religion has been distorted by Christian theological assumptions.

For those who employ an emergence narrative as a diagnostic tool, the cure is clear: scholars must slough off remaining theological fetters and develop rational methods for attending to phenomena other than those familiar to Christian intellectuals. When scholars succeed in generating rational theories and methods, the analysis continues, they will be able to recognize the contributions made by dancing and other bodily and aesthetic expressions to the life of religion.

While a number of scholars have made excellent progress in expanding the methods of religious studies to account for the physical and aesthetic dimensions of religious life, in so far as they espouse an emergence narrative of the field, they bump up against an unforeseen obstacle. Many of these efforts approach instances of dancing as one other object to which they apply their existing models and methods of analysis. They approach dancing as what Asad calls a "symbolic representation."[9] They do so as a condition of understanding it in a way other than that represented by "theology," where theology signals belief in some sacred or supernatural power. Such examples may be found across the field in studies of ritual as practice and performance, material culture, and popular religion. Catherine Bell, for instance, approaches ritual action as having a "vocabulary."[10] Susan Foster calls dance a form of "bodily writing."[11] Richard Schechner, in an effort to resist the textualization of religious phenomena, interprets the movements of Kathakali as "being written in the bodies of dancers" and "read" by them "from the inside."[12] In such cases, scholars

often resist as "theological" or "ideological" the participants' interpretation of what bodily actions accomplish. The obstacle is this: in
the effort to resist a theological interpretation (and thus attend to
bodily movement), scholars employ and reinforce a distinction
between "dancing" and "writing" that marginalizes dance within the
terrain of "religion."[13]

The problem is that we have yet to understand fully the forces that
drive textualization in religious studies. While I agree that the privilege accorded to verbal media by scholars of religion in their choice of
objects, methods, and goals does function, as Foucault says, to bury,
disguise, and disqualify dance as religion, it does not follow that all of
the forces authorizing this privilege can be attributed to the lingering
effects of Christian theological bias. Some indeed can. However, the
key impediment to considering rhythmic bodily movement as religiously effective is not, I argue, theological influence. As important,
paradoxically, is the *hostility towards theology*—what Catherine Bell
describes as the "nearly paranoid degree of antitheology polemic"[14]
—perpetuated by emergence narratives themselves. As this book
demonstrates, it is allegiance to an emergence narrative that drives
scholars to seek protection from theological infection by relying on
the practice of writing as a model, metaphor, and disciplinary method
for generating objective scholarship.

ANTITHEOLOGY POLEMIC

Evidence that adherence to an emergence narrative generates
"antitheology polemic" is present in the current polarization of the
field of religious studies. In general, "theology" functions as a roving
signifier for whatever appears to threaten the academic status of
scholarship in "religion." In this capacity, theology has come to have
at least two contradictory meanings: first, a belief in an essence or
core of religion that cannot be reduced to verbal or rational forms, and
second, a belief in rational method as capable of guaranteeing objec-

tive perspectives on religious phenomena. On the one hand there are social scientists committed to forging universally applicable, scientifically justified methods capable of *explaining* religion; on the other, there is a more diverse group of historians, phenomenologists, and social theorists committed to *interpreting* or *understanding* the particularities of a given religious complex or phenomenon. Representatives of each camp accuse those in the other camp of being too "theological," and for each camp, the hostility towards theology expresses a similar fear: that scholars will import some foreign element into their research (whether abstract formula or personal bias), project that element onto the phenomenon in question, and thereby lose the object they intend to investigate. Suspicion of theology polarizes the field.

In response, under pressure to distinguish what they do from "theology," scholars modern and postmodern, of social scientific and humanist bents, rely on tools of scholarship generated in the seventeenth- and eighteenth-century Enlightenments.[15] They deploy, as a primary line of defense, a belief that the practices of reading and writing serve to develop human reason into a free, mature faculty, operating over and against the corrupting forces of either "theology" or bodily experience. In studying "religion," scholars look for the kind of phenomena they know how to represent in words.[16] By trafficking in words, they can submit findings to a process of grading and review, and find validation in relation to other writing in the field. For representatives of either antitheology position, then, it is the concern for justifying their insights over and against theology that cements a commitment to linguistic models of interpretation, structures of explanation, and practices of training.

Where it is a scholar's concern for rational scholarship—her antitheology polemic—that fuels her commitment to writing, the implications for attending to dance as religion are more difficult to discern. From this perspective, inattention to dance is not accidental but *intrinsic* to the project of studying "religion." Adherence to an emergence narrative of the field hinders attention to forms of religious experience and expression that do not resemble writing in form or function. In short, where the impetus forging scholars' allegiance to verbal paradigms of knowing is an *antitheological* climate, the solution is not for scholars to complete an emergence of the field from theological influences, but to move beyond a conviction that "theology" represents the nemesis of academic study. Scholars interested in the study of religion and dance must find ways of delineating a flexible distinction between religion and the study of it that does not depend upon hostility towards "theology." When this development occurs, scholars of religion will be able to develop theories and methods of studying religion accountable to dance.

THEORIZING RELIGION AND DANCE

Towards the goal of acknowledging dance as religion, van der Leeuw points a way. Van der Leeuw offers a phenomenological analysis of religion and dance that remains, to this day, prescient across the fields of dance studies and religious studies. In Part 2, I examine van der Leeuw's perspective and the dynamics that influenced him in developing it.

Although van der Leeuw's interest in religion and dance was shared by others in his time, his insights were and remain unique. As van der Leeuw was growing up, signs of shifting attitudes towards dance as religion among mainstream Protestant cultures were appearing. In particular, Europeans witnessed the success of two forerunners of modern dance, Isadora Duncan (1878-1927) and Ruth St. Denis (1879-1967).[17] In the first decade of the twentieth century, each of these two American women performed, lectured, and taught, touring through the intellectual centers of Western Europe. For the first time in the Christian West if not in history, *women*, performing dances of their *own creation*, were appearing in *public*, *alone*, on a theater *stage*, claiming to *communicate* intellectual and religious *meaning*. Moreover, both women drew choreographic inspiration from traditions in which people danced their religion—Duncan from ancient Greece, St. Denis from Hindu, Egyptian, Buddhist, Hebrew, and eventually Christian traditions.[18] The dancing of these women catalyzed Christian and scholarly interest in dance. Ethnologists and historians of religion, as well as aestheticians and theologians took note. Van der Leeuw in particular credits Isadora Duncan with helping him name and understand phenomena that he witnessed in his historical studies of Greek, Egyptian, and Asian religions, in Islam, Judaism, and even in Christianity: historical moments in which "dance" appears in the "guise" of "religion." As he writes: "I shall mention with honor the name of the person who for the first time revealed to us the majesty of the dance, and that is Isadora Duncan."[19]

By the time van der Leeuw published the 1932 edition of *Wegen en Grenzen* (later translated as *Sacred and Profane Beauty: The Holy in Art,*) a steady stream of books on dance in history, anthropology, and theology had begun to appear.[20] In 1923, Oesterley completed his study of dance in the texts and cultures of the Hebrew Bible.[21] R.R. Marrett wrote that primitive religion was not thought or written, but *danced* (1932).[22] Musicologist Curt Sachs compiled his *World History of the Dance* (1937)[23] appearing alongside art historian Gertrude Kurath and anthropologist Franz Boas as three pioneers in the field of dance ethnology.[24] In 1938 Johan Huizinga issued his *Homo Ludens: A Study of the Play Element in Culture*, identifying dance as the "purest form of play."[25] In Christian contexts, meanwhile, Margaret Palmer Fisk laid out a biblical, historical, and theological defense for the inclusion of dance in Christian worship.[26] Louis Backman rehearsed the history of dance in Christianity.[27] By 1958, proponents of sacred dance—including Ruth St. Denis and her husband Ted Shawn—were gathering to establish the Sacred Dance Guild.[28] Even Paul Tillich, in the third volume of his *Systematic Theology*, acknowledged that Protestantism, in relation to the early and medieval churches, "has fallen very short of their creative power in all the visual arts, including those in which hearing and seeing are equally important, as in religious dance and religious play."[29]

Although van der Leeuw's interest in dance and religion was inspired and influenced by such developments in culture, scholarship, and religious studies, he nevertheless accomplished what no other scholar, theologian, or dancer has done since: he presented a compelling case for how and why the action of "dancing" can appear as religiously effective. There are books by Christian writers seeking to overcome a presumed antithesis between religion and dance.[30] There are pamphlets, articles, and books providing practical advice on how to defend and incorporate dance in Christian contexts.[31] There are a number of monographs that feature dance as it appears in the context of a given culture or tradition. Further, the last thirty years have witnessed a surge in publications in dance history, dance theory and dance anthropology, though few of these books pay attention to religion or to the work of religious studies scholars when illuminating the social, cultural, or psychological significance of dance.[32] Still, no one has picked up van der Leeuw's project of developing conceptual resources for theorizing coincidences of religion and dance.

No one has continued van der Leeuw's project, partly because the influence in religious studies of the emergence narrative since his death has diverted scholars from addressing the dynamics that give rise to a perception of religion and dance as mutually exclusive— namely the reliance on the practice of writing as a guard against theological bias. As van der Leeuw was aware, any attempt to welcome dance as an object of religious studies or an integral part of a Christian service must first dismantle the perception of an opposition between the two. Otherwise, "dance" can appear as "religion" only in so far as it conforms to a definition of religion predicated on the exclusion of dance. Dance, then, cannot appear.

What appears in van der Leeuw's work, however, is even more intriguing. He offers resources for rethinking the relationship between theory and theology in religious studies, but he also offers conceptual tools for thinking about dancing as religion. His work demonstrates how attention to dance as religion can catalyze innovations in our understanding of "religion," as both a category and as particular phenomena.

In reviving Gerardus van der Leeuw as a thinking partner, I challenge those who have evaluated his work through the lens of an emergence narrative as insufficiently liberated from theological bias. Scholars have accused van der Leeuw of assuming a mystical essence of religion; of embarking upon a "cultural crusade" to defend religion against its critics; of offering an "unintelligible" method for his phenomenology of religion, and of failing to account for his own Christian bias.[33] In short, van der Leeuw has appeared as a foil against which scholars on both sides of the antitheology debate vent their antipathy towards "theology" and defend their scholarly integrity.

In the hurry to move beyond van der Leeuw and towards a more rational footing, however, scholars of religious studies have failed to appreciate his contributions to the very concerns that impel them to dismiss him as too theological. Van der Leeuw designed his phenomenology of religion as a method for acknowledging and negotiating tensions between the study and practice of religion, between theory and theology. While affirming that scholars of religious studies can and will never "free" their project from "theology," he does not assume that theological perspectives can or will exist in harmony with scholarly interpretations. Rather, he embraces as necessary and generative a tension between religious studies and theology. He advocates a system of checks and balances that can guide scholars beyond the fear of theology that drives an overzealous allegiance to verbal expressions of authority.

The critique of the emergence narrative is underway. The time has come to continue what van der Leeuw began. We need a theory of dance in relation to religion that refuses to posit an essential or constant nature of dance or religion, and that seeks to understand the conditions under which a given person in a given time or place might experience rhythmic bodily movement as effective in relation to what he knows as religion.

CHAPTER OUTLINE

The following breakdown of Parts 1 and 2 into chapters is designed to orient the reader to the work to come. While my argument unfolds through the book as a whole, some readers may be eager to skip to chapters that deal directly with dance before fleshing out the enabling context of these reflections. Along the way, as I am writing for a group of readers that spans multiple disciplines, I keep the narrative as unencumbered as possible, gathering references to secondary literatures in the endnotes.

The four chapters in Part 1 examine a handful of seminal works in Christian philosophy and theology spanning the seventeenth to nineteenth centuries selected for their ongoing influence within emergence narratives of the field. Together, these chapters demonstrate that hostility towards "theology" represents a common strategy for negotiating an instability inherent within the project of studying "religion" itself. That tension, I argue, arises between the desire to *affirm* religion as a distinctive human activity, worthy of study, on the one hand, and the desire to provide an objective *critique* of religious thought and practice on the other. The works consulted here, albeit in different and mutually illuminating ways, all reject (some definition of) *theology* as a threat to the balance between critique and affirmation they seek to strike; all rely on the act of *writing*, as an ideal and as a practice, to authorize their perspective. In so far as these thinkers privilege writing as a hedge against the dangers of theology, they divert attention from dance as religion.

Chapter 1, "The Rift in Religion," traces these moments of affirmation and critique to a distinction between reason and experience that Enlightenment thinkers borrowed from the natural sciences as a foundation for developing theories of religion. Focusing on René Descartes and Immanuel Kant, this chapter comments on the ways in which each man uses the term "religion" to affirm *as rational* an idea or belief that he confirms *cannot* be proven through rational means. In their respective accounts of religion, "theology" stands for that which must be rejected in order to ensure this critical affirmation of religion. It is Kant in particular who inaugurates the move emulated by most scholars in religious studies to this day: he relies on the practice of writing as a method for resisting the seductive effects of theology. One implication of his strategy for stabilizing the study of religion is that dancing, and bodily expressions of religion in general, can appear only as derivative of religion's rationally-defensible core. Kant's strategy for negotiating a critical affirmation of religion remains paradigmatic in the field, even as the configurations of reason and experience, religion and theology, which he calls upon writing to secure, have evolved.

Chapter 2, "Recovering Experience," demonstrates how Schleiermacher's early critique of Kant's theory of religion further cements a resistance to considering dance as religion. In his classic, *On Religion*, Schleiermacher contends that the relationship Kant presumes between reason and experience is inadequate to negotiating a critical affirmation of religion. Schleiermacher, in response, uses the term "religion" to name a kind of "experience" that gives rise to reason and cannot be represented by reason—a feeling and intuition of the universe. Theology, in turn, represents for him a claim to truth whose fixity occludes ongoing receptivity to "religion." Finally, as this chapter argues, even though Schleiermacher reverses Kant's privileging of reason over experience, he continues to rely on the practice of writing to protect his account of reason and religion from theology. Thus, Schleiermacher's response to Kant further instantiates the idea that religion and dance are mutually exclusive activities.

Chapters 3 and 4 offer comparative analyses of G.W.F. Hegel and Søren Kierkegaard in response to issues raised by Kant and Schleiermacher. These chapters illustrate how Hegel and Kierkegaard draw distinctions between the science of religion and the practice of religion in ways that rely upon and reinforce a perceived opposition between dancing and writing.

Chapter 3, "Doing the Work of Spirit," describes Hegel's effort to reformulate the relationship between reason and experience, and on this new ground develop a "Science" or philosophy of religion capable of securing a critical affirmation of "religion." Embracing the perspectives he identifies in Kant and Schleiermacher, Hegel conceives of the relationship between reason and experience as a dialectical movement, progressing through history towards "Absolute Knowing." He names this movement "spirit." Chapter 3 explains how Hegel uses his concept of spirit to ground a Science of religion that is both objective (i.e., free from theological bias) and empathetic (i.e., attentive to the particular) in its reflections on religion. He does so by conceiving of religion and the Science of religion as two distinct yet interdependent moments that are reconciled in the dialectical movement of spirit. For Hegel, moreover, philosophical writing, defined over and against theology, is the practice through which that reconciliation between religion and the scientific study of it occurs.

In Chapter 4, "The Poet and the Dancer," a dancer appears as Kierkegaard's figure for what Hegel's Science cannot grasp about religion. For Kierkegaard, Hegel's Science cannot ensure the reconciliation of religion with the Science of it because no reason, no matter how dynamic, can understand the kind of experience—the leap—that faith is. This chapter focuses on *Fear and Trembling* to investigate why Kierkegaard describes his model of faith, Abraham, as a dancer. Kierkegaard contrasts dancing with philosophical writing to signal an unbridgeable chasm between religion and the Science of it. Dance appears as a metaphor for a dialectical relationship between reason and experience whose terms are held together only in the passion of a singular individual. Chapter 4 concludes that Kierkegaard's response to Hegel enforces a sense of opposition between writing and dancing as practices. In doing so, Kierkegaard helps elucidate the connection between adherence to an emergence narrative of the field and a difficulty acknowledging any contribution dance can make to theory and method in religious studies.

A conclusion to Part 1 argues that the contemporary desire to emerge from theology is suspect: it suggests an unwillingness to confront an irreparable fault at the heart of "religion." Emerging from theology has come to mean reducing or resolving the moments of critique and affirmation to one side or the other. Method-driven explanations of religion develop the critical moment over and against an affirmation of belief and experience. Interpretive approaches designed to preserve the particular timbre of religious voices develop the affirmative moment over and against critical attempts to explain religion away. By identifying these moments of affirmation and critique as integral to the study of "religion," Part 1 illuminates why a movement in either direction is defined by those who make it as a movement *away* from theology and decried by those who move in the opposite direction as *too* theological. It also illuminates how adherence to an emergence narrative reinforces a belief in the practice of writing (as model, method, discipline) and thus undermines attempts to acknowledge dance as effective in relation to religion.

In Part 2, I turn to the work of van der Leeuw. Writing a half-century after Kierkegaard, van der Leeuw works out another strategy for securing a critical affirmation of religion, one that does not demonize theology nor reinforce an opposition between dancing and writing to secure objectivity. Van der Leeuw does so by embracing affirmation and critique as moments in a rhythm that generates the field.

Chapter 5, "A Braided Approach to the Study of Religion," introduces van der Leeuw's braided methodological approach to the study of religion as one that casts a role for theology in the study of religion. He advocates incorporating theology as a critical, contested voice in the project of understanding religion. In his fluid and dynamic model, the disciplines of theology, phenomenology, and history of religions (including both social scientific and humanist approaches) appear as distinct yet interdependent projects. They check and balance, compel and constrain, fund and correct one another. In the process, as Chapter 5 explains, the relationships among the disciplines enact a dynamic, dialectical relationship between reason and experience that preserves moments of affirmation and critique as comprising a paradox which is generative of (understanding concerning) "religion." It is van der Leeuw's braided approach, I contend, that enables him to resist both the lingering theological paradigms and antitheological polemics within the field that deflect scholarly attention away from dance as religion, and enforce a perception of writing in opposition to dancing.

Before exploring van der Leeuw's phenomenological renderings of religion and dance, Chapter 6, "A Practice of Understanding," digs more deeply into van der Leeuw's phenomenology of religion in order to excavate what he means by "phenomenon" and what he recommends to a phenomenologist interested in understanding it. For van der Leeuw, a phenomenon is simply "what appears," and the job of the phenomenologist is to recreate the conditions that enable a given phenomenon to appear to her or him by practicing skills of imaginative empathy, intellectual restraint, and a constant oscillating attention between the folds of her own experience and knowledge and the stuff of history. In short, the task of the phenomenologist is to cultivate his ability to move back and forth between reason and experience, history and theology, form and chaos, and thereby cultivate his receptivity to appearances of meaning.

Chapter 7, "Understanding Religion and Dance," explores the renderings of religion and dance which van der Leeuw generates through his own practice of understanding. From his perspective, phenomena that appear as "religion" appear as expressions of "power" or "holiness"; phenomena that appear as "dance" appear as impressions and expressions of "beauty" through movement. With these perceptions, van der Leeuw sets the stage for identifying coincidences of religion and dance in the historical record as conveyed by historians of religion and evaluated by theologians. Under what conditions, he asks, does a phenomenon conduct at once an experience recognized as both "dance" and "religion"?

Chapters 8 and 9 lay out a rich array of conceptual paradigms that van der Leeuw offers scholars and dancers who are interested in such coincidences. These chapters provide the resources needed to lift dance into view as an integral, contributing element of religious life. Chapter 8, "Spanning the Unity of Life," focuses on the first of five "structural relations" or conceptual nets van der Leeuw employs in order to capture coincidences of religion and dance. Here, dance appears as religion in so far as dance appears to enact the "unity of life." Chapter 8 explores the numerous paradoxes or rhythms nested in this claim along two axes: dance as body and dance as culture. Chapter 9, "Marking Boundaries," explores four other appearances of dance and religion van der Leeuw identifies, ranging from conflict to harmony.

In a conclusion to Part 2, I summarize the implications of these chapters. By approaching coincidences of religion and dance through his mediating phenomenological practice, van der Leeuw is able to comprehend the apparent antithesis of dance and religion embedded in the study of religion as a function of a "structural" or "comprehensible" association connecting those phenomena that appear as "dance" and those appearing as "religion." In the process, he resists both the theological bias against dance fueled by a lingering Protestant paradigm, and the antitheological ignorance of dance as a nonverbal and thus naive medium of religious life. His work suggests that writing and dancing are interdependent modes of knowledge, equally implicated in the study of religion. Through these expositions, the value of van der Leeuw's method for the contemporary study of religion appears.

Chapter 10, "Dancing Religion," entertains a discussion of why attention to dance as religion is important for scholars of religion, and what implications such attention may have on the evolution of theory and method. Where the perception of dance as an adversary of religion may have facilitated the formation of the field, the continuing vitality and relevance of the study of religion will require attention to dance as religion. In this process, dance is both a phenomenon to consider and a resource in the development of theory and methods capable of attending to it. I conclude with an agenda for future projects in the philosophy of religion and dance.

Part One
WRITING AGAINST THEOLOGY

An analysis of Christian philosophers and theologians writing on the eve of the so-called emergence of religious studies from theological contexts reveals a dynamic not predicted by emergence narratives of the field. Early modern Christian philosophers and theologians introduce "religion" as a category in generative tension with "theology" as competitors in a project of Christian reform.[1] Emergence narratives to the contrary, it is difficult to find a moment in the modern era when a project of theorizing "religion" exists in cooperative, congenial intimacy with "theology," even when the thinker in question is a professed theologian.

Part 1 revisits the work of five thinkers whose reflections on religion remain authoritative in order to lay the groundwork for an alternative narrative of the field. The current double designation of theology (as an overreliance on either method or essence) points the way. This double designation may be traced to two contradictory moments embedded in modern uses of the term "religion" as a category for rational reflection and analysis. As I discuss in detail below, each of these thinkers employs a distinction between reason and experience authorized by the successes of scientific discoveries in seeking to provide a theory that both *affirms* and *critiques* what they describe as "religion." They seek a theory capable of affirming as religion claims to truth whose authority derives from sources other than reason, while at the same time assessing the value of such claims in relation to the needs and capabilities of free reason.

Although these thinkers offer diverging definitions of religion, the primary strategy they all employ to negotiate the contradiction inherent in this project is to distance their perspectives from "theology" and call upon the practice of writing as a primary line of defense. Theology appears most often to represent a claim to truth that cannot be verified by rational reflection on the contents and conditions of lived experience. As such, theology threatens to topple the precarious balance between critique and affirmation to one side or the other, either by supporting a theory of religion insufficiently distinct from the phenomenal or doctrinal forms of religion (and losing the critique), or by presuming to evaluate the merits of any given religious phenomenon on some ground other than its own (and losing the affirmation). In either case, theology augurs a loss of either an objective purchase on religion or an ability to appreciate the particular forms of religious life as *religious*. From the perspectives offered by these thinkers, it is difficult to appreciate dance as anything other than one of those particular forms whose value derives from its ability to serve the development of reason.

In the double designation of theology, then, lies an inkling of an alternative to the emergence narrative of the field—one promising a different fate for theology, for van der Leeuw, and in turn, for the study of dance and religion. When the history of the study of religion is remembered as a series of attempts to articulate and stabilize this tension between affirmation and critique, the story appears as one of an ongoing *generative tension* between theory and theology rather than as one of *emergence from* theology. From this perspective, theory and theology are ever engaged in a relationship whose inevitable friction generates new versions of each. The rift between affirmation and critique cannot be wished away or smoothed over. It poses an ongoing challenge to scholars of "religion."

The narrative of generative tension offered in these chapters elucidates the relationship between moments of affirmation and critique represented by each thinker's use of the term "religion." It traces the changing shapes of this relationship, details the role played by writing in sustaining this relationship, and illuminates the implications of particular choices for considering dance as religion. In this narrative, "theology" appears as a critical voice, a perspective upon which scholars call to assess whether or not they succeed in striking an enabling balance. Within this narrative, moreover, "dancing" appears alongside writing as a metaphor and model for religion. As Chapter 4 elaborates, it is Kierkegaard who first discerns this possibility when he calls upon the image of dance to characterize the faith of Abraham. In short, the matrix of issues unfolded in Part 1 opens to reveal a relationship between dancing and writing at the heart of modern Western attempts to theorize religion.

In revisiting these early voices, then, Part 1 narrates a pre-history of the field designed to encourage scholars to invest their imaginative energies in futures other than that represented by an emergence from theology—futures more amenable to the consideration of dance as a medium of religious experience and expression. If there was no Eden-like harmony of interests between theology and theory at the origins of the field, there can be no pure *telos* of distinction into which the field is emerging. Part 2 will demonstrate how attention to dance as religion in particular can provide scholars with resources for envisioning and realizing alternative futures.

CHAPTER 1

The Rift in Religion
René Descartes and Immanuel Kant

René Descartes (1596-1650) and Immanuel Kant (1724-1804), often considered as representing the respective ends of the European Enlightenment, each drew upon the methods of "science" in an attempt to clarify the nature and value of "religion."[1] They each were concerned with various excesses they observed among Christians in their time. Though most often remembered as ushering in distinctively modern uses of reason, Descartes and Kant were both equally concerned, as this chapter illustrates, with defending religion from what they perceived as reason's abuses. In hindsight, it is possible to see how choices these men make in negotiating this tension between critique and affirmation predict the fate of dance in the field of religious studies to date.

CHANGING SHAPES OF RELIGION AND SCIENCE

In the sixteenth and seventeenth centuries, when theological and institutional differences pitting Christians against one another exploded into a prolonged series of military conflicts, philosophers and theologians turned towards "science" to seek resources for advancing Christians beyond discord and towards the realization of Christian values and ideals. Science at this time was not a discipline distinct from mathematics or philosophy; the term was used to refer to such projects as well as to the natural sciences, a group itself not yet subdivided into biology, chemistry, and physics. The word "scientist" had not yet been coined.[2] Generally speaking, science included a range of projects loosely characterized by a common method of pursuing knowledge: practitioners of science exercised their reason in relation to the contents of their experience. Those engaged in science formulated hypotheses and designed experiments to help them gather evidence through their senses; they compiled measurements and lists of features, which were in turn made subject to classification and mathematical modeling. They sought to provide accounts of the natural world that could be tested, verified, and refuted through the repetition of experiments.

Moreover, as they pursued these tasks, practitioners of science did not maintain a clear distinction between science and Christian faith; they were most often Christians, and their belief in scientific method, their hopes for its outcomes, and their desire to participate in its success were frequently informed and sustained by Christian values. Some went so far as to perceive their work as a spiritual practice and an ethical directive demanded by their faith in God. As Francis Bacon (1561-1626) writes:

> Wherefore, if there be any humility towards the Creator, if there be any praise and reverence towards his works: if there be any charity towards men, any zeal to lessen human wants and sufferings; if there be any love of truth in natural things, any hatred of darkness, any desire to purify the understanding; men are to be entreated again and again that they should dismiss for a while, or at least put aside, those inconstant and preposterous philosophies which prefer theses to hypotheses, have led experience captive, and triumphed over the works of God.[3]

Appealing to his readers' sense of Christian virtue, Bacon demands that they perceive how their "experience" is held "captive" by claims to knowledge that are not based on methods of experiment and observation. It is by drawing "near to the book of Creation," Bacon admonishes, that readers may be washed clean of false belief, superstition, and unsubstantiated claims to knowledge. This book of Creation "is that speech and language which has gone out to all the ends of the earth, and has not suffered the confusion of Babel; this men must learn again, and, resuming their youth, they must become again as little children and deign to take its alphabet into their hands."[4] Science, in Bacon's hands, offers a method for liberating rational reflection on experience from the scourge of *theology*.

Attempts to read the appeals to Christian virtue in such apologies for science as mere utilitarian veiling assume a distinction between "religion" and "science" which had not yet crystallized. For Bacon and others, the practice of science promised to clarify people's relation to God and not only by liberating their experience of the natural world from inconstant philosophies. The ability of science to deliver results that were valuable depended upon belief in God: it is because nature is a *book*, that is *created*, and is *one* book, that humans can progress individually towards certain and true knowledge of the world through reflection on their own sensory experience. Science arises as a means for enacting the commensurability of reason, experience, and the natural world—a commensurability represented by the idea of God as All-knowing Creator. Science, moreover, enacts this commensurability by serving as a method of *reading and writing*: in science, humans develop their reason along the lines of its own God-given capacity by disciplining it through acts of hypothesis, experimentation, and observation to the designs of God's Book. By attending to their sensory experience of the natural world, then, practitioners of science believed they were exercising and fulfilling their capacity for knowing. In this way, they perceived their successes in amassing knowledge of the natural world as bearing witness to the one God, Creator and Sustainer of all.

For philosophers and theologians concerned with mediating the strife among Christians on the cusp of the modern era, the *content* of scientific discoveries was less interesting than the philosophical *ground* which the successes of science appeared to prove: namely, the distinction between reason and experience. As Kant later describes the situation, what "all students of nature" learned from Galileo, Torricelli, Stahl, and others is that reason has the capacity to serve as an "appointed judge" over the contents of sensory experience, compelling its observations and the results of its experiments to yield answers to its questions.[5] Where reason is honed as an ability to articulate the *sense* of sensory experience, then, scholars inferred, if properly trained and applied to Christian history, scripture, and tradition, reason might serve to liberate the human relation to God from unsubstantiated theologies.

As we shall see in the cases of René Descartes, Immanuel Kant, and those after them who operate within the paradigm of knowledge their works describe, the scientific method has value for the study of religion indirectly—not as a method for gathering knowledge about *God* per se, but rather as a model for acquiring knowledge about the *physical* world that scholars may then consult in the process of developing rational methods for acquiring knowledge about *metaphysical* issues, involving freedom, the soul, immortality, and God.

In particular, these two thinkers adopt as the basis for their inquiries into religion the distinction between reason and experience authorized by the successes of science in reading the natural world. They mobilize "religion" as the name for those doctrines, practices, and institutions that lay claim to a knowledge that cannot be verified by reason on the basis of empirical authority. Because they predicate their theories on the ability of reason to attain knowledge through reflection on experience, the problem of what humans can and cannot know about "God" lies at the heart of their projects. If reason secures knowledge through reflection upon the contents and conditions of experience, then what can reason know about an eternal, absolute infinite, unbound by time and space that is not an object of experience? Can reason arrive at a knowledge of God that may be verified independently of the idiosyncrasies of a given denominational cast? Descartes and Kant seek to identify a rational core of religion capable of drawing Christians together across denominational lines as members in a common body of Christ. As we shall see, the manner by which these men resolve the problem of what humans can know about God, though different, serves to exclude dance from consideration as contributing to the value of religion so defined.

ENLIGHTENMENT ENDS

René Descartes is an example of one who had hope for the clarity that the paradigms of science could bring to the project of Christian reform.[6] His search for "the true method of obtaining knowledge of everything which my mind was capable of understanding" takes as human, and as given, the ability to distinguish reason from experience.[7] In seeking a method capable of leading him to a first principle or starting point in relation to which all other principles and knowledge may be referred, he uses his "reason" to dismiss the contents and processes of his sensory experience. As he reports in his *Discourse on Method*, his first principle is: "never to accept anything as true unless I recognized it to be evidently such" for "reason obliged me to be irresolute in my beliefs" (12, 15). Describing his method of refusal or doubt in his *Meditations on First Philosophy*, Descartes writes,

> I shall consider myself as having no hands, no eyes, no flesh, no blood, nor any senses, yet falsely believing myself to possess all these things; I shall remain obstinately attached to this idea, and if by this means it is not in my power to arrive at the knowledge of any truth, I may at least do what is in my power . . . and with firm purpose avoid giving credence to any false thing. (M 62)

Descartes' doubt is not all encompassing. It does not extend to the distinction between reason and experience, or to the capacity of reason to dismiss the contents and processes of sensory experience.

Convinced that sensory engagement with the world produces contra-dictory perspectives on what counts as certain and true knowledge, Descartes decides to place his hope in reason based on its scientifically verified ability to rise above and reflect upon experience.

By his own account Descartes spent "nine years" practicing the art of detaching his reason from his experience, "trying everywhere to be spectator rather than actor in all the comedies that go on" and living "in appearance, just like those who have nothing to do." (DM 18,19). Eventually in Holland, in the midst of war and winter, he found a warm, quiet room. There, enjoying "all the comforts of life to be found in the most populous cities while living in as solitary and retired a fashion as though in the most remote of deserts," Descartes' method proved its worth. He arrived at an end and a beginning of cer-tain knowledge:

> I soon noticed that while I wished to think everything false, it was necessarily true that I who thought so was something. Since this truth, *I think therefore I am*, was so firm and assured that all the most extravagant suppositions of the skeptics were unable to shake it, I judged that I could safely accept it as the first principle of the philosophy I was seeking. (DM 21)

By means of a method in which he *practices* distinguishing reason from experience, Descartes discovers his "self" as a "a thing which thinks . . . which doubts, understands, [conceives], affirms, denies, wills, refuses, which also imagines and feels" (M 66). He discovers his self as a power to distrust all sensorially mediated impressions. In this discovery, reason reflects on itself, affirms its capacity for self-reflection, independent of the mediating influence of experience.

In turn, when viewed through the lens of this first principle, Descartes perceives other elements of his existence, including his embodiment, as accidental to his essential self:

I then examined closely what I was, and saw that I could imagine that I had no body, and that there was no world nor any place that I occupied, but that I could not imagine for a moment that I did not exist . . . therefore I concluded that I was a substance whose whole essence or nature was only to think, and which, to exist, has no need of space nor of any material thing. Thus it follows that this ego, this soul, by which I am what I am, is entirely distinct from the body and is easier to know than the latter, and that even if the body were not, the soul would not cease to be all that it now is. (DM 21)[8]

Here, the content of Descartes' discoveries confirms the techniques of his method. While he does not deny that he is a body, he affirms that he has an ability to imagine himself without one. It is because he can imagine this absence that he feels justified in asserting that the locus of his agency, autonomy, and reflective capacity is "entirely distinct" from "body."[9]

On the basis of his ability to imagine a clear distinction between reason and experience, soul and body, Descartes concludes that he is more certain that God exists than that he has a body.[10] Reflecting back onto his years of practicing doubt, Descartes interprets his need for such a journey as evidence that "my spirit was not wholly perfect, for I saw clearly that it was a greater perfection to know than to doubt" (DM 22). Searching for some "source" from which he could have "learned to think of something more perfect than myself" he arrives at the following "hypothesis": "that this idea was put in my mind by a nature that was really more perfect than I was, which had all the perfections that I could imagine, and which was, in a word, God" (DM 22). Descartes' God, then, appears as the author of an idea of perfection, an idea that manifests itself in Descartes as a felt dis-ease with the unreliability, the perspectival, ephemeral nature, of sensory experience. Reflecting on his sense of disappointment with experience as a ground for knowledge, Descartes deduces the existence of a greater perfection

responsible for that disappointment. As an idea, Descartes' God justi-
fies his suspicion of experience and, at the same time, ensures that his
practice of detaching his reason from experience is what will enable
knowing of what is. Through such detachment, a reasoner comes to
know God with certainty as unifying or theorizing the disparate contents of sensory experience. Although Descartes first comes to know
his self as double, what he finds in reflecting upon his self is an eternal, pre-existing unity of God.[11]

For Descartes, this hypothesis of God as eternal perfection provides
the litmus test for evaluating all knowledge about God, and all forms
of religion—including theology—in which that knowledge is embedded.[12] For example, he writes, "doubt, inconstancy, sorrow and similar things could not be part of God's nature"; God has no "corporeal
nature" since "intelligent nature is distinct from corporeal nature"
and "composition is an evidence of dependency and that dependency
is manifestly a defect" (DM 23). "Religion," in turn, appears as a category to affirm critically that subset of Christian teachings and practices that support his rationally derived idea of God. Through the
practice of his method, then, Descartes arrives at an idea of God
whose form and content justify his starting point—the freedom of
reason to reflect on itself over and against the processes and contents
of sensory experience.

The readiness with which Descartes dispenses traditional forms of
his Catholicism in the quest for certain knowledge about God leads
some critics to question his personal faith and religious commitments. For such readers, Descartes marks the threshold of modernity:
he discards religion in favor of science, initiating the slow emergence
of science as an authority over and against religion in general, and
theology in particular.

However, by focusing on Descartes' use of the distinction between
reason and experience, a second interpretation is possible in which
Descartes' orientation to the forms of his tradition expresses his
commitment to "religion." By predicating his idea of God on his abil-

ity to imagine that he has no body—that is, his ability to enact the power of reason over sensory experience—Descartes provides a rational ground for affirming the value and necessity of an idea of God that he hopes may facilitate understanding and agreement among Christians, and by extension, other peoples. Where God is an idea generated by reason's reflection on itself, and not an object one must experience, then all people, regardless of their embodied circumstances, can potentially know "God" with certainty as their source. All people can know God because all people can imagine themselves as existing independent of their bodies. Rather than dismissing Christianity, then, Descartes may be read as wielding a theory of religion that allows him to affirm and critique its theological claims about what lies beyond the reach of embodied sensory experience based on the ability of those claims to express and encourage the freedom of reason in its pursuit of eternal perfection, harmony, and love. In this reading, Descartes' rational idea of God appears in competition with theology over the fate of religion.

This alternate reading of Descartes' method thus reveals a rift in the term "religion" that, while assuming various guises since, finds expression in the current antitheology polarization among members of the field today. Where the litmus test for religion is an idea (of God) whose authority rests on the ability to imagine one's body as absent, scholars evaluating a phenomenon as "religion" make two diametrically opposed conceptual moves. First, they affirm that the particular sensory forms comprising "religion" carry a distinct and recognizable meaning for someone; and second, they base the affirmation of those sensory forms on the degree to which those forms serve an idea of God as that which is universally inaccessible to sensory experience. Both moves are now criticized separately as evidence of theological bias: presuming rational method over and against religious phenomena and assuming the existence of a God or a sacred as the essence of religion.

While such an imaginative act is possible to perform and often useful, when used as a basis for theories of religion, it carries myriad implications for what can and cannot appear as religion—such as dance. Before analyzing these implications, however, attention to Kant's theory of religion serves to flesh out the links connecting attempts to negotiate the two moments of affirmation and critique with a suspicion of theology that seeks relief in practices of writing.

NEGOTIATING THE RIFT IN RELIGION

In a number of ways, Immanuel Kant continues Descartes' project, drawing upon the distinction between reason and experience authorized by scientific discovery to develop a theory of religion. Writing at the far end of the Enlightenment, however, he is concerned that scholars, in their enthusiasm over the powers of reason, have claimed more for reason than reason can justify. He faults Descartes, for example, for assuming that the ability of a human to conceive an idea of perfection means that such perfection must exist. According to Kant, at the moment Descartes claims knowledge of a supersensible Being that he cannot justify on the basis of experience, he speaks with the voice of theology. Kant's response is to bind reason more tightly to the realm of experience—without losing the distinction between them—and thus foreclose the possibility of any knowledge, mediate or immediate, about God (CPR 82).

The irony is that less becomes more. By limiting reason to what it can know from experience, Kant makes a stronger case for why "religion" is necessary and inevitable in human life—and for why human reasoners must constantly engage and critique religion, including the forms of Christian history. By recasting the relationship between reason and experience Kant endeavors to negotiate the rift in religion and balance the moments of affirmation and critique. He wields the term "religion" to slice away those symbols, ideas, and practices within Christianity that do not support the process of reason's reflection on experience, while affirming, at the heart of Christianity, a "religion" occurring "within the limits of reason alone." The points of this argument are spread across several of Kant's works. This chapter gathers them together, introducing ideas Kant lays out in his *Critique of Pure Reason* (1781), and tracing their application to questions of religion through two classic essays, "An Answer to the Question: What Is Enlightenment?" (1784) and "What Is Orientation in Thinking?" (1786) as well as his later *Religion within the Limits of Reason Alone* (1793). In the process, I highlight how Kant relies upon the practice of writing to stabilize his theory of religion in relation to "theology."

REASON'S EXPERIENCE

"Experience," in Kant's view, refers to the realm of sense perception. It is an active mesh that seizes and receives impressions, a mesh that both connects and separates the faculty of reason—as the locus of human agency, the "I," the capacity for self-reflection—from the universe. All that a reasoning "I" can know is derived from processing the information conveyed through one's particular sensory sieve; by first, classifying its contents (the process of understanding), and then distilling from those classifications general principles of relationship (the process of reason). Correlatively, Kant surmises, human reason can never attain certain and true knowledge about the world "out there" or even of the objects that appear to it, for reason can never reach around the categories of time and space that enable a person to experience that world in the first place. A person knows an object only as it appears to her; she cannot know that object as it appears to someone else, or as it is "in itself." For Kant then, as humans receive no sensory evidence of God, reason cannot *know* God, nor know anything about God: "There can be no doubt that all our knowledge begins with experience" and "God" is not an object of sensible experience (CPR 41).

Even so, as for Descartes, Kant does allow for the possibility that reason can attain knowledge about *itself* by reflecting on what must be true in order for reason to experience and understand at all. Such knowledge "begins with" experience, though it does not "arise out of" experience, for it represents knowledge of what "our own faculty of knowledge . . . supplies from itself" (CPR 41-2). Such is the realm of pure reason Kant discusses in his first *Critique*. It is in this space of reason's self-reflection, or reflexivity opened up by the presumed distinguishability of reason from experience, that Kant delineates the right and the need for individuals to reject the traditional forms of Christian theology and establish a personal, rational relationship to God.

First of all, as Kant summarizes in his essay, "What Is Enlightenment?", where there can be no irreducible points of authority that reason can discern outside of the demands of its own operation, then reason is justified in rejecting all claims to uncontestable truth made in human history by others.[13] Where there can be no knowledge of the absolute, there can be no grounds for claiming absolute knowledge.

Moreover, not only are human reasoners justified in suspecting all claims to supersensible knowing, but to the extent that reason is this power, a reason that has not interrogated such claims suffers from "self-incurred immaturity." In so far as people adopt as true "dogmas and formulas" which base their claims on supersensible realities they forestall the maturation of their reason in its capacity to detach itself from experience, reflect upon it, and derive knowledge. "Dare to know!" Kant pleads, counseling his readers not to rely on the advice of others in making decisions about what to believe and how to act: "*Immaturity* is the inability to use one's own self-understanding without the guidance of another."[14] The case is especially true in "matters of religion." As he writes, "religious immaturity is the most pernicious and dishonourable variety of all" (WE 59). Any contract to abide by "a certain unalterable set of doctrines," Christian or otherwise, when concluded with a view to preventing all further enlightenment of mankind forever, is absolutely null and void, even if it is ratified by the supreme power, by Imperial Diets and the most solemn peace treaty. One age cannot enter into an alliance on oath to put the next age in a position where it would be impossible for it to extend and correct its knowledge, particularly on such important matters, or to make any progress whatsoever in enlightenment. This would be a crime against human nature, whose original destiny lies precisely in such progress. (WE 57)

The process of "enlightenment" demands that a person exercise and thereby realize the freedom of his reason over and against sensory experience by holding all forms of knowledge—including and especially religious forms—accountable to what can be known through sensory experience. By contesting theological claims, a reasoner demonstrates his ability to distinguish his own reasoning activity from the forms of knowledge (such as religious doctrines) mediated to him through sensory experience. Not even the "most solemn peace treaty" is more important than this practice.

Kant goes further: not only does he employ the distinguishability of reason from experience as justification for urging his reader to throw off the "ball and chain of his permanent immaturity" (WE 55), he claims for reason the authority to determine what in human experience qualifies as "religion." Because there are no grounds outside of sensory experience on which to anchor a "permanent religious constitution" (WE 58), the conditions required for the free operation of reason themselves appear as the sole criteria for evaluating doctrines, teachings, practices of religion. To demand that a person surrender her ability to "extend and correct" knowledge is to "nullify a phase in man's upward progress"; it is an act equivalent to "violating and trampling underfoot the sacred rights of mankind" (WE 58). "Matters of religion" that do not honor, encourage, and further this "sacred right" do not warrant attention; they not only may, but must be discarded. The ultimate point of accountability in the definition and evaluation of religion is the process of enlightenment itself.

What then can a reasoner who practices and preserves his freedom in the pursuit of knowledge know about "God"? What value does Christianity have for one whose reason is enlightened? Even though Kant denies that any claims to knowledge can ever *be* absolute, he nevertheless affirms that humans need ideas *about* the absolute. Sometimes, Kant admits, reason is called upon to make judgments about things that extend beyond the realm of what a person can deduce from experience through understanding and reason. In such instances, reason feels a "need" for a compass, an idea of an absolute, in order to orient thinking. In this "feeling of a need which is inherent in reason itself," Kant finds a toehold for *rational belief* in God as comprising the core or essence of religion.[15] This "feeling of a need" is not a sensation that arises in (sensory) experience, but rather represents reason's perceptions of its own kinesis and of the conditions required for its own reflective, reflexive activity.

According to Kant this orienting concept assumes the shape of "God" in response to two felt needs: theoretical and practical. First, a person seeking to gather knowledge through an analysis of experience feels a need for an idea of a perfect, unlimited creator, an overarching order of creation, as a context for explaining the contingent existence of everything limited (WO 241). The project of classification, Kant attests, is a process of referring limited phenomena to a larger order and as such, presumes as its condition some overarching "purposiveness" within which a particular moment may appear as having a meaning which can be named and explained. Yet there is no object in our experience capable of serving this end. He writes that "in order to explain the phenomenon in question, reason needs to presuppose something which it can understand; for nothing else to which it can attach a concept is able to remedy this need" (WO 242). Without such an assumption of purposiveness, the project of explanation is impossible and pointless.[16] Here Kant articulates what the earlier apologists of science allowed: the project of science—and its authority in demonstrating the distinction between reason and experience—presupposes an idea of infinite Being capable of ensuring that what reason is capable of discerning through experience corresponds in some measure with what is. Nothing in human experience guarantees this commensurability.

In addition to this theoretical need, reason also feels a practical need—a need that arises in its attempt to formulate moral laws (WO 242).[17] Kant is adamant that reason does not need an idea of God to authorize moral law, nor to provide motivation for abiding by the moral law, whether as a promise of reward or threat of punishment. As he insists in *Religion within the Limits of Reason Alone*: "morality does not need religion at all."[18] Humans obey the moral law because by doing so they preserve the conditions needed for the free maturation of their reason. The reason is given by reason. Reason as well postulates the existence of God in order to give "objective reality to the concept of the highest good" (WO 243). Kant observes that because humans have a propensity to wonder about the outcomes of their actions, they will derive more *pleasure* from obeying the moral law if they have some concept of the end to which their obedience is leading—some vision of absolute goodness, the "highest good." "Without an end of this sort," he writes, "a will, envisaging to itself no definite goal for a contemplated act, either objective or subjective (which it has, or ought to have, in view), is indeed informed as to *how* it ought to act, but not *whither*, and so can achieve no satisfaction" (RLR 4). To serve this purpose of "satisfaction" in action, reason authorizes a belief in a "whither"—the idea of God, as a "higher, moral, most holy, omnipotent Being," who ensures that the ends of my moral action will contribute to realizing eventually the "highest good" in the world (RLR 4-5).

In response to these felt needs of reason, Kant supports a concept of "God" that gives "objective reality" to the existence of an infinite Creator and absolute Good. This concept must be true for the healthy exercise of reason in its pure and practical functions. Justification for believing in the existence of a supersensible, eternal "God" rests firmly on the felt needs of reason: "The *concept* of God and even the conviction of his *existence* is to be found only in reason as its exclusive source" (WO 245). Neither claims to revelation or personal experience, nor appeals to Church, Bible, or Tradition can override the authority represented by the needs reason feels in its efforts—its sacred right—to expand and correct its knowledge about the world and about its responsibilities for action within the world. Correlatively, as Kant confirms, a rational belief in God is one that can never be transformed into *knowledge* that would justify its imposition on another human reason (WO 244). Rational belief is by definition a place to which all humans must journey on their own in the process of enlightening their own reason.

Despite his focus on rational belief as the essence of religion, Kant does not dismiss all phenomenal forms of religion. Once thinkers arrive at a rational ground for belief in an idea of an absolute infinite Being, this concept of "God" provides them with a path back to the historical, theological forms of religion that they necessarily rejected in the process of maturing their reason. According to Kant, rational belief provides a "touchstone of reliability," an "ultimate touchstone of truth," for claims concerning what lies beyond the realm of sensory experience (WO 243, 249). As he writes, "a purely rational belief is the signpost or compass by means of which the speculative thinker can orient himself on his rational wanderings in the field of supra-sensory objects" (WO 245). All claims to miracles, revelation, human nature, God's existence, and so on that support both the content *and* the process of coming to rational belief earn the designation "religion"—a "religion within the limits of reason alone." Only when humans acknowledge that they can never know God with certainty through the sieve of sensory experience are they able to postulate an *idea* of God, *believe* in the existence of God, and *practice* religion in a way that preserves the freedom and maturity of their reasoning faculty. Rational belief in God can serve as a path to the historical forms of religion because and only because it is a form of conceiving God that remains solely beholden to the free development of reason.

Not only does Kant endorse his idea of a rational belief in God as providing practitioners of Christianity with a method for appropriating religious doctrine and practice, he also asserts that such an idea provides the framework and the necessary condition for a *"philosophical* theory of religion" (RLR 10). Scholars can evaluate the "history, sayings, books of all peoples, even the Bible" according to the criteria of rational belief (RLR 8). By starting "from some alleged revelation or other" as an *"historical system"* and then seeing "whether it does not lead back to the very same pure *rational system* of religion," scholars can identify, compare, and contrast historical systems which allege revelation based on the degree to which those systems align with the needs of a maturing human reason (RLR 11). Thus Kant appeals for a new discipline, arising alongside "Biblical theology" with "religion" as its focus.

TWO MOMENTS, EXPOSED

In Kant's theory of religion, the two moments of affirmation and critique activated with every application of the term religion appear in full form. On the one hand, when Kant names as "religion" a given "historical system" of ideas, institutions, artifacts, practices, stories, texts, etc., concerning supersensible realms, he affirms that complex as a distinct element of human life with a role to play in nurturing the enlightenment of human beings. On the other, such a complex appears as valuable through a process of selection in which those facets that mirror a rational belief in God are privileged and others set aside. In other words, the process through which scholars identify some set of claims and practices as "religion" is the same process through which they evaluate those claims as not certain and true on their own terms, but only in so far as they correspond to a rational belief in God wielded by the mature reason of an observer.

These contradictory movements in turn arise as a direct result of the way in which Kant presumes and defines the distinguishability of reason and experience as the basis for his theory of religion. On the one hand, a scholar succeeds in generating a theory of religion only in so far as she is able to secure the freedom of her own reasoning activity from attachment to doctrines claiming knowledge of super-sensible, "unalterable" truths. Only when she is convinced that she cannot know God through her experience, that God is absent from all experience, that all human claims to knowledge of God are thus sus-pect, will she maintain the freedom needed to *critique* different claims and practices concerning supersensible knowledge based on the ways in which they serve the enlightenment of her own reason. By this approach, a scholar is predisposed to notice as "religion" the kinds of phenomena whose claims to truth she suspects.

On the other hand, Kant appeals to this same distinction of reason from experience to *affirm* that the forms of religion against which reason exercises its critical freedom are nonetheless an essential (and ever-contested) component of human life. Because human reason is limited in what it can know to the contents and conditions of sensible experience, humans necessarily construct concepts and practices to help them orient their thinking about what lies beyond the reach of their sensory experience. Here, paradoxically, Kant's reasoning human is not free: he cannot claim freedom from his own need for a rational belief in God without falling prey to dogmatism and fanati-cism of all kinds (WO 248). Thus, any attempt to critique phenomena of religion on the basis of a rational idea of God affirms the necessity of supersensible claims that it nonetheless exposes as not equivalent to knowledge.

In sum, where the definition and meaning of the term "religion" presume the relation of reason and experience as articulated by Kant, scholars applying the term mobilize a paradox, at once affirming the importance and inevitability of the cultural forms whose claims to supersensible truth they simultaneously contest. Every act of naming a historical system alleging revelation as religion affirms both the historical system as a response to the human need for postulating supersensible realities and, because those constructions will never grasp "God," the need to interrogate constantly the ability of those constructions to nourish the continuing activity of reason in making them.[19]

RESISTING THEOLOGY

In Kant's attempt to negotiate these two moments of affirmation and critique, shades of the contemporary hostility among scholars of religion towards theology appear. For Kant, "theology" as a claim to supersensible knowledge is suspect. In so far as theologians assume the existence of God and speak as if they know with certainty the nature of God, they tempt maturing reasoners to seek refuge from the hard work of developing their own rational relation to the absolute. If human reasoners claim to *know* God with certainty, their reason destroys itself by renouncing the very condition of its operation—freedom. They lose their ability, their willingness, their justification, and their criteria for evaluating religion. In so far as they privilege their own tradition as representing absolute truth, they cannot affirm another historical system as a rational system of religion; instead, it appears in comparison with their truth as merely false. Concomitantly, if they cannot affirm historical phenomena as religion, neither can they critique them based on their ability to support the enlightenment of human reason. Thus, the freedom and flexibility to wield the term religion as an affirmative and critical perspective on the alleged revelation of historical systems demands that scholars resist the temptation to surrender their reason to any particular religious constitution.

At the same time, however, Kant's suspicion of theology is not anti-religion. To the contrary: the suspicion of theology protects the balance of critical and affirming moments involved in theorizing religion not only by preserving a scholar's freedom from the claims of theology, but as importantly, by preserving the philosopher's personal *connection* to her tradition. A scholar's suspicion of theology ensures that her relation to her own tradition—its theology included—will be mediated by her reasoning activity—and by her understanding of it as "religion," that is, as a rationally defensible system. In this way, a scholar's suspicion of theology guides her in developing a relation to her own tradition—and its theology—that is not vulnerable to the claims of other traditions but is rather affirmed by her critique of those other forms. She is able to appreciate the authority of her own tradition based on the way it manifests the character shared by all systems whose alleged revelations enable rational development: the felt needs for rational belief. In other words, for Kant, only in so far as a scholar acknowledges her own need for rational belief, can she effectively name, appreciate, and evaluate religions, including her own, as species of rational belief.

Concomitantly, if Kant's suspicion of theology is not anti-religion, neither is it intended to be anti-Christian. By balancing the affirming and critical moments involved in theorizing religion, and by guarding the freedom of reason in its distance from and relation to the forms of religion, Kant's suspicion of theology represents his attempt to participate in the progress of his own Christian tradition. His suspicion of theology expresses what his concept of rational belief leads him to identify as the core of the Christian message—the need for individuals to exercise their own reason in their journey to rational belief in one absolute, eternal, good God. In the end, Kant's suspicion of theology does not even appear as anti-theology, per se, but rather as a guide to conceiving and doing theology in ways accountable to the exercise of humans' "sacred right."

THE PRACTICE OF WRITING

In his attempt to deflect the influence of theology over maturing minds, Kant recommends a strategy that remains a model for scholars in the contemporary study of religion. He advocates the practice of writing for a reading public. For Kant, it is through the practice of writing that people exercise and enact the freedom of their reason over and against experience—including their experience of theological claims regarding knowledge about God.

In defending the right of maturing reasoners to write, Kant introduces a counter-intuitive distinction between the public and private uses of freedom. Citing the examples of military personnel, taxpayers, and then clergy, Kant denies that individuals are entitled to a "private use of freedom." In the civic roles and responsibilities that individuals assume, "obedience is imperative" (WE 56). Theologians, in particular, when hired as clergy, are obligated to prioritize "care for the soul's welfare" over scholarly concerns (RLR 7). By contrast, the freedom Kant advocates as necessary for enlightenment is the "freedom to make *public use* of one's reason in all matters . . . that use which anyone may make of it *as a man of learning* addressing the entire *reading public*" (WE 55). Public freedom is the freedom to read, think, and write, and to do so in the privacy of one's study; it is the freedom to argue, to question, and to contest all authority, to comment upon the "inadequacies of current institutions" for the purposes of advancing the process of enlightenment in all realms—scientific, political, religious, etc. (WE 57). For Kant, then, the practice of writing represents the mental, physical, and emotional space in which a person exercises his capacity to detach his reason from the contents and processes of his sensory experience and reflect critically on them. In writing, humans enact—or make real for themselves—the ability of reason to reflect critically on civic responsibilities, familial relations, and religious affiliations. For Kant, then, writing serves as a practice of freedom—a discipline through which people sense, exercise, and lay claim to their sacred right to critique claims to absolute knowledge.

At the same time, as writing persons demonstrate for themselves the inadequacy of all forms of human knowing, they confront their own limits as well. As we have seen, it is through this process of exercising freedom in relation to theological dogma that human reasoners clarify their felt need for (a concept of) God. A reason disciplined by the act of writing develops an awareness that its strength and apparent autonomy derive from its ability to assess and analyze the contents and processes of experience. It is as people work out their criticisms of theological claims in writing, with a reading public in mind, that they come to sense and appreciate their own need for an orienting belief. They mature their reason to the point where they can justify their belief based on the felt needs of reason, and thus justify their use of rational belief as a theory of religion—a universally applicable category for evaluating particular historical systems alleging revelation.

In this way, the discipline of writing performs for Kant a function akin to that provided by the act of imagining that one has no body for Descartes. In both instances, a person rehearses the conditions that must be true in order for her to find a rationally defensible relation to "God" at the heart of "religion." As Kant insists, "the *public* use of man's reason" is "all that is needed" for enlightenment (WE 55).

IGNORING DANCE

Within such approaches to theorizing religion, a lack of attention to dance is not an accident. There has been no mention of dancing in this chapter because the orientation towards religion assumed by Descartes and Kant inhibits the process of recognizing dance as religion.[20] Where the project of naming, comparing, and evaluating religion proceeds by wielding either an idea of God as the eternal absolute, or a rational belief in God as infinite truth and goodness, both inaccessible to sensory experience, in either case, then, in so far as "dance" refers to the experience of performing physical movements, it can figure as only ancillary to the work of religion. Dancing registers as meaningful and valuable in so far as a scholar can recognize it as contributing to the process of reason's enlightenment.

Correlatively, this lack of attention paid to dance as religion cannot be fully explained by recourse to a lingering Protestant bias towards rational and verbal modes of religious experience and expression, in opposition to physical, sensory modes. Neither Descartes nor Kant encourages hostility towards human bodies. On the contrary, they each embrace sensory immersion in experience as a source of knowledge. For Kant in particular, human reason remains accountable in what it can know to the conditions, processes, and contents of sensory experience. While each thinker practices detaching reason from experience, the need to practice such detachment is evidence of the interdependence of reason and experience. Further, the freedom reason secures through such practice is a freedom from being determined by the phenomenal forms of experience, not an absolute freedom. Reason remains accountable in what it can know to the evidence provided by sensory experience.

Descartes and Kant, in fact, are both committed to locating the rationality of religion in relation to human embodiment—in relation to the concerns and challenges of life in an empirical world. It is because they embrace this goal that religion appears as a problem in the first place—as a set of historical systems whose norms, values, and truth claims do not appear, at least initially, to serve the cause of a reason that dwells in and through human bodies. The reason these thinkers ignore dance, then, is not that dance is "body" as opposed to "word" per se. Rather, imagining dance as religion would confuse the distinction between reason and experience that Descartes and Kant strive to *realize* as the necessary condition for mounting a critical defense of religion. One can imagine them thinking that dance either represents an activity in which reason directs the actions of "the body," thus adding nothing to what reason can know, or conversely, an activity in which the power of sensory experience sways and informs reason, perhaps enough to confuse its reflections on experience. In either scenario, dance would fall short of the criteria required to serve the maturation of reason.

Further, while Descartes and Kant do privilege verbal forms of expression as conduits of rational analysis and meaning, their purpose for doing so is intrinsic to this project of providing a critical affirmation of human religion. For Kant in particular, writing enacts both the critical distance from and the empathetic, rational relation to the phenomena at hand. His appeal to the practice of writing as a condition for reason's maturity acknowledges that writing affects the way in which people think—not just the objects that they notice, but the way in which they orient their thinking and engage with the material at hand. What is more important to the neglect of dance then, than the value accorded to verbal media or rational expressions of religion per se, is the reliance on writing as a disciplinary practice. A person who practices writing as a means for exercising and confirming the freedom of reason from determination by sensory experience cultivates an ignorance of the ways in which embodied experience enables and informs his or her rational capability.

The critique of enlightenment reason as disembodied is as old as the pietist and feminist voices of the Enlightenment and as new as feminist and postmodern work in the 1990s.[21] The problem highlighted here is not a distinction between reason and experience (sometimes reified as the mind/body problem), but the way in which thinkers conceive that distinction as natural or given and use it as a ground for knowledge. As critics discussed in the next three chapters advance, Descartes and Kant develop only one facet of that relationship in cultivating a sense of reason's freedom from determination by experience. While it *is* possible to train human beings to think in these ways and generate insightful understanding of religious phenomena in the process, this style of engaging religious phenomena serves to highlight aspects of religious life that mirror a scholar's writing practice (in privileging reason over experience) as those which are most relevant to the meaning and value of religion. To contemplate the idea that dancing may itself represent a medium of knowledge would require theorizing other facets of the relationship between experience and reason, as well as of the relationship between religion and the study of it. The next three chapters begin this work by examining critiques of the enlightement paradigms as represented by Descartes and Kant in the writings of Friedrich Schleiermacher, Hegel, and Kierkegaard.

Before investigating further the implications for dance of these Enlightenment paradigms for theorizing religion, I turn to the critique of Descartes and Kant leveled by Kant's contemporary, Friedrich Schleiermacher. Schleiermacher's response will serve to highlight those features of their projects that discourage attention to dance as religion.

CHAPTER 2

Recovering Experience
Friedrich Schleiermacher

In his address to the "cultured despisers" of religion, Friedrich Schleiermacher (1769-1834) was speaking, among others, to admirers of Kant. First published in 1799, six years after Kant's *Religion within the Limits of Reason Alone*, Schleiermacher's *On Religion: Speeches to Its Cultured Despisers* openly rejects Kant's attempt to negotiate a critical affirmation of religion. Schleiermacher's response is most often remembered as defining a pole diametrically opposed to Kant's rational defense: Schleiermacher elevates a particular kind of inner experience over and against rational belief as the locus of religion.[1] Nevertheless, as the following close reading of *On Religion* suggests, his difference from Kant serves to reinforce similarities between their projects as well, including dynamics inherited by scholars in the study of religion that to this day hinder attempts to acknowledge rhythmic bodily movement as an effective dimension of religious life.[2]

The critique of Kant Schleiermacher advances in *On Religion* is one that he maintains, with various elaborations, throughout later theological works. He claims that attempts to define religion as a rational system reduce religion to questions of metaphysics and morals.[3] The "religion" they project is dead. As such, he avers, these approaches are incapable of affirming the meaning that religious phenomena have for people. Schleiermacher insists that, regardless of intent, an approach like Kant's tips the balance of affirmation and critique too far to the side of critique. For those inclined to despise religion, Kant's picture confirms what they want to believe: religion is unnecessary and even harmful for the free maturation of human reason.

Even so, in orchestrating his alternative theory of religion, Schleiermacher does not dislodge the distinction between reason and experience assumed by Kant. As explained below, he relies on his conception of this distinction in order to strike an enabling balance between the moments of critique and affirmation inaugurated by any use of the term "religion." In doing so, Schleiermacher, like Kant, maintains a suspicion of theology and finds in the practice of writing a protective strategy. As such, Schleiermacher's difference from Kant reinforces dynamics in the field of religious studies that foreclose attention to dance as religion.

EXPERIENCING THE UNIVERSE

Investigating the reasons for Kant's failure to produce a theory of religion that is both affirming and critical, Schleiermacher targets Kant's conception of the relationship between reason and experience. While Schleiermacher concurs with Kant, Descartes, and those who share their view that humans may cultivate their reason as a self-reflective, thinking faculty over and against the sway of sensory experience, he faults Kant for failing to appreciate the double movement in the relationship of reason and experience that Kant's account of this relation implies. Where Kant emphasizes a scholar's ability to reflect upon sensory experience as the factor enabling her rational belief in God and thus her study of religion, he locates religion in a vector moving from reason to experience. In so doing, he ignores the role played by the vector of influence moving in the converse direction—from experience to reason. As Schleiermacher points out, the bounds that Kant claims experience places on reason imply this second direction, and here, he insists, is where we find "religion." Staking out his difference from Kant and others, Schleiermacher writes, "Religion's essence is neither thinking nor acting, but intuition *and* feeling. It wishes to intuit the universe, wishes devoutly to overhear the universe's own manifestations and actions, longs to be grasped and filled by the universe's immediate influences in childlike passivity."[4] We are far from rational belief.

In understanding the significance of this quotation for discussions about dance, the "and" is the key. For one, by naming religion as a matter of intuition *and* feeling, Schleiermacher is not only defining religion in opposition to thinking and acting, he is defining religion as a kind of experience that is inaccessible to reason. For Schleiermacher, "intuition" and "feeling" represent the component parts of one moment called "religion" that appear to reason only in hindsight, in distinction from one another, as what was fused in that moment. "Feeling" refers to an inward sensation of being moved, being impressed, or having been encountered; "intuition" refers to a mental picture of whatever that moving, impressing something must have been. Feelings represent the subjective remnants—the felt sense of "I"—and intuitions represent the objective remnants—a sense of an "it"—of what was, for a flash, one indivisible experience. Thus, in defining religion as intuition and feeling, Schleiermacher stretches Kant's category of experience to include not only the sensory input upon which a reasoning "I" reflects, but a sensory engagement out of which reason itself emerges as a remainder. Religion *is* the union of what in reason is divided; it names a dimension of human existence that cannot appear in consciousness as an object through a process in which a subject detaches his sense of "I" from, and reflects upon that object. Religion thus eludes reason not because religion represents a claim to knowledge concerning a supersensible Other (as some critics of Schleiermacher assert), but rather because it is a moment of sensory engagement with the universe in which the distinctions between reason and experience, thinking and sensing, do not apply.[5] "Religion never appears in a pure state" (21); it appears only in the shape of a memory, as a longing for that which is absent—that is, as a feeling attached to, yet separated from an intuition.

While every sensory experience may leave traces of its passing in intuitions and feelings, those intuitions and feelings characteristic of religion carry distinguishing marks: they appear as "of the universe."As Schleiermacher asserts, religion appears in consciousness as a devout wish to "be grasped and filled by the universe's immediate influences." The feelings associated with religion include feelings of infinity, majesty, awe, humility, freedom, agency, and love; the intuitions of religion include those that reach to represent a whole or eternal generative matrix giving life in every moment.[6] Schleiermacher is clear: there is no Object out there distinct from a human subject to which these feelings and intuitions correspond. The feelings and intuitions of religion are representations, fragments left in the wake of an experience of sensory immersion in and continuity with a greater creative activity. God, he explains, is simply the name of one intuition that humans invent to represent to themselves the cause of their feelings: "whether we have a God as part of our intuition depends on the direction of our imagination" (53). Given this understanding of religion as the feeling and intuition of the universe, then, any theory of religion which proceeds by divorcing feeling from intuition and evaluating the latter as a rational system misses the connection to feeling that gives intuitions their meaning for someone as traces of an experience which has passed and can never be present. Taken apart from the feeling content, Schleiermacher insists, any intuition, including "God," is "empty mythology" (25).

In insisting on the internal relation between feelings of boundless totality and intuitions of eternality, Schleiermacher introduces another aspect of his critique of Kant: religion is embodied and contextual. Religion marks an experience so singular and irreducible that at that moment it *is* all that is. Listen as Schleiermacher describes the "natal hour of everything living in religion": "I lie on the bosom of the infinite world. At this moment I am its soul, for I feel all its power and its infinite life as my own; at this moment it is my body, for I penetrate its muscles and its limbs as my own, and its innermost nerves move according to my sense and my presentiment as my own" (32). In religion, a person's senses enter and fill with the world as she experiences her relation to some object, landscape, piece of music, or person as being all that is. Finite self and infinite source interpenetrate: she is its soul; it is her body. In such a moment, a person does not perceive herself or the catalyst-object of her experience as a *part* of an "infinite world," nor as a *microcosm* of a whole, nor as existing in any causal or derivative relationship to a whole. As Schleiermacher confirms, "religion . . . stops with the immediate experiences of the existence and action of the universe, with the individual intuitions and feelings; each of these is a self-contained work without connections with others or dependence upon them" (26). In religion the singular *is* infinite. The eternal *is* embodied. As Schleiermacher intones: "Those who truly know about their religion and its essence will utterly subordinate to the particular every apparent connection and will not sacrifice the smallest part of the particular to it. The realm of intuition is so infinite precisely because of this independent particularity" (27). By implication then, theories of religion that try to represent religion through concepts such as part, whole, human, absolute, infinity, good, and their logical relations abstract intuitions from bodily experience and lose religion. Such theories surface after a particular moment of religion in response to it as a way to remember in general terms what occurred.

Where religion is "feeling and intuition" of the universe inaccessible to reason, embodied and particular, implications follow for a different system of education to religion than that proposed by Descartes or Kant. For Schleiermacher, the ability to understand and appreciate religion requires awakening a "sensibility and taste for the infinite" (23): "Without our faculty of sense no universe is found" (61). Schleiermacher explains: "there is implanted in each person his own drive to allow every other activity to rest for a time and only to open all sense organs in order to let himself be penetrated by every impression. Through a secret, most beneficial sympathy, this drive is strongest when universal life reveals itself most distinctly in one's own breast and the surrounding world" (60). This capacity to "open all sense organs" is one that "approaches" objects and "offers itself to their embraces"; it "strives to grasp the undivided impression of something whole. It wants to perceive what and how something is for itself and to recognize each in its unique character" (61). It is a faculty of sense, Schleiermacher argues, whose maturation requires discipline, namely, practice in stilling the kind of engagement with the world which treats sensory impressions as raw material for digesting into knowledge. "Prudent and practical people," he insists, are "robbed of their faculty of sense" by their need to accomplish goals and produce results; sensory awakening, by contrast, requires "comfortable inactive rest."[7] Thus, by naming religion as the intuition and feeling of the universe, Schleiermacher implies that attempts to affirm religion as a rational system fail not only because they separate intuitions from feelings, but because they represent an exercise of reason that ignores the conditions enabling reason's rational reflection on religion. For Schleiermacher people seeking to understand religion must use their reason to enhance their receptivity to experiences of the universe that will stretch and pull them into new shapes of intuition and feeling. Understanding religion is not about withdrawing from the world into mystical or rational abstraction. Rather, we can know religion only by cultivating constantly an open sensory awareness that suffuses all thinking and acting—including our thinking about religion. Schleiermacher intones, "religious feelings should accompany every human deed like a holy music; we should do everything with religion, nothing because of religion" (30).

It is in describing the sensory awakening and reorientation of reason which understanding religion entails, that Schleiermacher makes his signature appeals to inwardness and depth. He extols: "I wish to lead you to the innermost depths from which religion first addresses the mind" (10); he calls his readers to attune to the "depths of the heart" (13), and find religion springing "necessarily and by itself from the interior of every better soul" (17). Yet, in making these appeals, Schleiermacher is not suggesting that the experience of religion is inner as opposed to outer, or emotional as opposed to rational, or even immediate as opposed to mediate as some commentators claim. Such distinctions are the province of reason, not religion. Schleiermacher's point is rather that religion *includes* that most inwardly felt sense of an "I" that reason supports. For Schleiermacher, reasoning persons cannot pursue knowledge about "God" or truth without feelings of infinity, freedom, and agency, and without intuitions of wholes comprised of parts. Nor can they formulate and legislate moral laws concerning the Good without feelings of respect and appreciation for particulars, or without intuitions of each particular as a whole in itself. While these religious feelings and intuitions do not determine the content of knowledge nor the forms of the moral law, respectively, they nevertheless fund the desire to know that propels reason towards maturity; they stir people's willingness to abide by the self-legislating activity of their own reason (23). In this sense, then, Schleiermacher stresses the inward depths from which religion springs in order to emphasize his point that religion does not exist as an entity from which people can detach themselves in order to reflect upon and evaluate the merits of its service to (inner) reason. It is religion that first "addresses the mind" and not the other way around. Said otherwise, moments of religion always already express a human capacity for sensing bodily being as dwelling in energetic interpenetration with the uninterrupted, ever-revealing, "ever-fruitful womb" of the universe (25).

Here Schleiermacher rests his case with the "cultured despisers": not only does their enlightenment quest for freedom, truth, and tolerance through a process of maturing human reason require religion, but in shaping and pursuing those goals, the cultured despisers of religion inadvertently presume religion and already practice it. In the felt needs of reason which Kant identifies as the ground for rational belief, Schleiermacher sees evidence that a mature, enlightened human reason presumes a person's sensory openness to feeling and intuiting him or herself as (partaking in) the ceaseless generativity of the universe.

TWO MOMENTS, PRESERVED

Readings of Kant and Schleiermacher that map differences between their theories of religion in terms of reason versus feeling, or mediated versus immediate experience overlook the similarity and thus the difference of Schleiermacher's position. As is evident in *On Religion*, Schleiermacher embraces the terms of Kant's project. He too intends to generate a theory of "religion" which is capable of providing rationally defensible criteria for both affirming the value of historical systems alleging revelation—including Christianity—and critiquing their excesses. He too adopts the distinction between reason and experience as a philosophical premise and, despite locating religion in the reverse direction of influence—from experience to reason—he opts for similar strategies in defending his preferred balance of critique and affirmation. He rehearses Kant's suspicion of theology and his reliance on the practice of writing as a strategy for defending his theory of religion from theology. Implications for attending to dance as religion follow in step.

First, as with Kant, Schleiermacher's critical intention is evident: he concurs with his readers that "religion" is worthy of scorn and derision as an "old folk-costume" for the lower classes (10), an "empty and false delusion" (12) that feeds fanatical violence and intolerance among humans. At the same time, his stated intent is to help his readers perceive and affirm the sparks of "religion" in these forms. To understand religion is to read these forms as *representations*, that is, intuitions of the universe, which have been misunderstood by practitioners as well as by despisers of religion as *claims to knowledge*. Perceived as claims to knowledge, the forms of religion are inadequate. Perceived as catalysts for stirring and awakening an ongoing sensitivity to new feelings and intuition, they may be highly effective.

Schleiermacher further confirms that this ability to read the phenomenal forms of religion as calcified intuitions depends upon a scholar's ability to free her reason from the particular representations of experience that lay claim to her allegiance. Here, his position aligns with Kant's again: a scholar's ability to sustain the freedom of her reason from experience is essential for maintaining her own connection to religion as the context out of which her understanding of historical systems alleging revelation can emerge. Where for Kant, the space between reason and experience preserves a person's freedom to arrive at rational belief, for Schleiermacher, this space preserves a person's vulnerability to be grasped at any moment by an awareness of the ceaseless gifting of the universe. A person must open a space between reason and (past representations of) experience in order to ensure that she remains open to reason-enabling experiences. In other words, a person's ability to see the phenomenal forms of religion as intuitions and feelings is crucial if she is to sustain a mature reason.

In this way, for Schleiermacher as for Kant, the practice of distinguishing between reason and experience provides both method and criteria for simultaneously *affirming* religion (as what reason needs in order to mature—whether rational belief or feelings and intuitions of the universe) and *critiquing* religion (based on whether its forms support the freedom and needs of reason in distilling or opening to experience). Even though Schleiermacher emphasizes a different vector of influence—moving from experience to reason—as the locus of religion, he nevertheless evaluates those experiences in terms of their service to reason. As he assures the cultured despisers, the feelings and intuitions he recognizes as religion advance enlightenment ideals of progress, knowledge, tolerance, and individual freedom.

Not surprisingly, it follows that Schleiermacher's commitment to mount a critical affirmation of religion also finds expression in a suspicion of "theology"—or at least, in a particular concept of theology. As Schleiermacher admits, he is a theologian "of the same order" as the persons his cultured readers despise. Nonetheless, echoing Kant's distinction of the private versus public use of reason, Schleiermacher insists that he is writing for a literate public as a human being: "Permit me to speak of myself" (8). In his *Speeches*, he claims to write through the crush of feelings and intuitions left in the wake of his own religion-experience and remember the pieces of these moments for others. He writes as a mediator not a theologian (7).[8] He writes in order to witness to a human capacity and need for religion, not to persuade readers to embrace a particular tradition as true. He implies that to speak as a theologian would upset the precarious balance between affirmation and critique required to understand and receive religion.

In this way, for Schleiermacher, as for Kant, scholars interested in providing a critical affirmation of "religion" fail if they cannot secure the freedom of their own reason from "theology." In so far as a theological claim seeks to bind reason to the particular intuition or representation of experience it represents, it collapses the distinction between reason and experience on which a critical, affirmative theory of religion hinges. For Kant, only a reason free to reflect upon theology is able to affirm the value of Christian tradition from a rational perspective, as an expression of rational belief—as a paradigmatic "religion." For Schleiermacher as well, only a person whose reason floats free from theological claims is able to sustain a responsiveness to subtle stirrings of sensory engagement with the world, preserve a respect and appreciation for particular moments of the generative universe, and thus develop her or his rational capacity to reflect upon another person's intuitions as expressions of a human longing for religion. Said otherwise, scholars' ability to arrive at rational belief (for Kant) or cultivate a vulnerability to religious experience (for

Schleiermacher), and in either case, appreciate these qualities in the phenomenal forms of historical systems alleging revelation, depends upon an ability to exercise reason in recognizing theology as one more phenomenal form of religion. When scholars do so, they preserve not only an objective perspective on "religion," but also the full flowering of their own "religion" as the necessary condition of that objective study.

WRITING STRATEGIES

Like Kant, in his attempt to protect his conception of the relation between reason and experience from theological distortion, Schleiermacher adopts as his primary strategy one that unwittingly encourages ignorance of dance as a medium of religious experience and expression. He invokes the *practice of writing* as a discipline in which a person exercises the capacity of reason to invite and reflect critically upon the intuitions and feelings of sensory experience.[9]

For Schleiermacher as for Kant, the practice of writing opens a physical, mental, and emotional space in which people can sense and make real for themselves a distinction between reason and experience as the enabling condition of their insights into religion. Recall that for Kant, writing provides a practice through which a person learns to critique all claims to knowledge (including and especially theological claims) and to confront his need for rational belief; as such, writing serves to mediate between a person's commitment to religion and his study of religion in a way that guarantees the health of the former and the objectivity of the latter. The practice of writing for a reading public ensures that the critical moment implied in naming a phenomenon "religion" will adequately represent the phenomenon so-named, and that the affirmative moment in turn will align with the needs of reason.

For Schleiermacher, the situation is similar: writing serves to mediate between a person's own connection to religion and her study of it so as to ensure both empathy and a critical perspective. Writing likewise accomplishes its mediating work by providing a person with the opportunity to enact the freedom of her reason from the intuitions and processes of experience—including those represented by theology. Writing marks the distance between Schleiermacher the theologian and Schleiermacher the human being. Yet, for Schleiermacher, the ability of writing to exercise the freedom of reason from experience serves reason *indirectly*: by writing, a person preserves the freedom of *experience* from determination by *reason*, and in this way, funds the continuing generativity of rational reflection. Schleiermacher embraces writing as a way to express what it is about religion that *eludes* rational representation. Schleiermacher is clear: his writing cannot make religion present. However, writing can provide him with a medium for reflecting upon his awareness of experiences of religion that have passed. In his writing, he distinguishes feeling from intuition in order to remember their thorough interpenetration at the moment of their conception; he contrasts religion with metaphysics and morals in order to highlight the interdependence of reason and religion. In and through writing, he can remember the component parts of those experiences and savor the changes in his sense of self and world wrought by their passing. By writing then, Schleiermacher guides his readers to cultivate their reason in ways that open their faculty of sense, that is, their capacity to be impressed by the ongoing gifting of the universe.

Further, writing about religion allows Schleiermacher, like Kant, to model an approach to his own particular religious tradition that is both critical and affirming. By identifying Christianity as a religion, he acknowledges that it constitutes only one set of intuitions among others. At the same time, he affirms Christianity as that network of intuitions, concretized in doctrines, texts, art, music, liturgy, and church communities, in which this picture of religion as the feeling and intuition of the universe emerges most clearly and decisively. He writes that Christianity "is none other than the intuition of the universal straining of everything finite against the unity of the whole and of the way in which the deity handles this striving, how it reconciles the enmity directed against it and sets bounds to the ever-greater distance by scattering over the whole individual points that are at once finite and infinite, at once human and divine."[10] In writing, then, Schleiermacher exercises the freedom of his reason to deny finality to any theological or rational intuition, and simultaneously affirms the intuitions of Christianity as fossils of an experience worth having. In writing, Schleiermacher demonstrates for his readers how he applies his concept of religion in ways that sustain his own rationally defensible openness to the gifting of religion through particular religious forms—in this case, Christian ones.

In Schleiermacher's view the value of writing for remembering religion and for modeling a critical, affirming approach to a tradition has corresponding values for readers as well. Schleiermacher holds open the possibility that his verbal descriptions may dislodge his readers' attachment to particular intuitions for *or* against religion, stir in them a desire for religion, and orient them in their pursuit of it. As illustrated by the passages quoted already, Schleiermacher milks the cadences, textures, and tone of his prose to incite readers' sensibility and taste for religion. He directs his readers' attention to spaces and surfaces of sensory awareness. By professing his inability to convey a moment of feeling and intuiting the universe, he piques his readers' curiosity about what potentials reside within them, beyond their ability to read his book. Schleiermacher begs his readers to find and awaken their own inner faculties for sensory engagement with the fruitful womb of the universe: "Become conscious of the call of your innermost nature, I beseech you, and follow it" (50). Given the kind of experience religion is—one that demands a conscious cultivation of sensory awareness—an "inmost" desire for it is requisite to having it. Thus, while Schleiermacher admits the inability of writing to transmit religion, he nevertheless uses writing to create the conditions necessary for an occurrence of religion in his readers.

Even so, Schleiermacher is well aware of the conundrum he inhabits: he is writing about what cannot be written. Pressed against the impossibility of his task, he interprets his urge to write about religion as further proof of the tenacity and undeniability of his experience. Driven by "the inner, irresistible necessity of my nature . . . that which determines my place in the universe and makes me the being that I am," he cannot do otherwise (5). Schleiermacher writes for a reading public, so he claims, because he must. He must express his sense of himself as a person opened and transformed by religion into someone capable of understanding and appreciating the meaning and value of apparently irrational manifestations of religious life.

For opposing reasons, then, both Schleiermacher and Kant rely upon the practice of writing to guarantee the successful deployment of the term "religion." They embrace writing as a practice that *enacts* the particular relationship between reason and experience on which their theories rest. Writing serves as a defense against those who would arrest either the kind of sensory experience that enables reason (for Schleiermacher) or the kind of reason that derives rational belief from an analysis of the contents and enabling conditions of experience (for Kant). For both then, writing ensures that the act of naming a phenomenon as religion will express a *free reason*—a reason that is neither attached to any one representation of experience as absolute nor in denial about its need for religion, and that neither uncritically embraces theology as "true," nor completely rejects it as "false." For each thinker, writing is the disciplinary practice that ensures that the study and living of religion can and will proceed hand in hand in a rationally defensible manner.

ROOM FOR DANCE?

At first glance Schleiermacher's account of religion as embodied and particular appears more congenial than Kant's in its potential for acknowledging dance as religion. One might argue that where religion entails an experience of sensory openness to the creative gifting of the universe, dance may serve as a practice of awakening and heightening a person's sensory awareness. However, Schleiermacher's commitment to writing as a practice for maintaining a proper relationship between reason and experience curtails this potential. For Schleiermacher, the practice of writing models and facilitates the kind of sensory awakening that yields a healthy reason, one capable of appreciating theological claims as calcified intuitions.

Correlatively, even though Schleiermacher does embrace a faculty of sense as the enabling condition of religion, his account of how to employ human embodiment in pursuit of religion discourages rhythmic bodily movement in favor, as noted, of "comfortable inactive rest." Here it is true that, in so far as Schleiermacher was informed by his upbringing and education in the pietist and enlightenment strands of modern Christianity, he had few examples of dance as religion from which to draw either in elucidating his theory of religion as an open sensory engagement or in executing a comparative project. Yet even if he had been exposed to Christians dancing, it is likely that his reliance on the practice of writing for maintaining a proper relationship between reason and experience would predispose him to discount them. The sensory awareness integral to religion, however privileged, still demonstrates its value in terms of the role it plays in enabling people to reason themselves free from phenomenal forms of religion. A person seeking to defend dance within such an approach to religion would need to argue how dancing is like a "holy music," accompanying and serving the needs of reason in the pursuit of metaphysics and morals.

In short, the largest obstacle to the consideration of dance as religion derives from how Schleiermacher assumes the distinction between reason and experience and relies on the practice of writing to protect and maintain it against the threat of theology. Where the project of theorizing religion involves distinguishing a rationally defensible core of religion (whether defined as rational belief or as a felt experience) from the phenomenal forms that express it, there is little chance that a phenomenon such as dance can appear on its own phys- ical, kinetic terms as religion. Again, the problem is not an association of dance with the body, sexuality, or women. Schleiermacher had a high if idealized regard for all of these. The obstacle to considering dance as religion lies in how writing is conceived and practiced as the model for organizing the relationship between reason and experience. In such an approach to religion, "dance" suffers a fate similar to "the- ology": its action appears as an external elaboration of religion, and not religion itself.

AN UNSETTLING LEGACY

In the contemporary scene, the positions represented by Descartes and Kant on the one hand, and Schleiermacher on the other, have come to represent opposing poles in the antitheology debates. Scholars fault theories of religion such as those of Descartes and Kant as too theological for over-privileging rational method at the expense of particular people, acts, and contexts. Theories like those of Schleiermacher are evaluated as too theological for over-emphasizing the irreducibility of religious experience at the expense of objective understanding. Across the field, a common theme reverberates: an objective study of religion cannot repeat these errors.

Yet, the examples of Schleiermacher and Kant, as recounted here, suggest that an emergence from theology (as they are defining it) is not a possible path to securing that objective study. For one, a resis- tance to "theology" as detrimental to the study of "religion" already comprises an integral, constitutive component of each man's efforts to theorize religion. "Religion" is designed as a hybrid, relational, reflexive term, emerging in stiff if cordial tension with theology, understood as claims to truth about "God." "Religion" appears as a check on theological thinking, but also as a call to develop a new way of thinking about, relating to, and even doing theology—a way that fosters the continued health of a rationally defensible core of religion that Schleiermacher and Kant define. "Theology" and "religion" appear in a conflicted but mutually generative interdependence. There is no original harmony.

What may prove more unsettling for contemporary theorists of religion about positions represented by Kant and Schleiermacher then, is not their theological moments per se but that they embrace what I am calling the rift between affirmation and critique as representing an irreducible paradox that is generative of *both* religion and the study of it. In theorizing religion, Kant and Schleiermacher assume the role of a conscience. They are goading their traditions to define themselves in line with those elements capable of making the most valuable contribution to the advancement of enlightenment ideals. To this end, they appeal to a scientifically valid distinction between reason and experience to define a core or essence of religion (as rational belief or inner experience) that provides criteria for evaluating phenomenal forms—including theology. In this sense, then, their efforts to theorize religion generate both critical perspectives *and* more religion as the necessary complements of one another. As such, critics attest, their theories are biased by their desire to coax into being the religion they desire.

Nevertheless, these thinkers do not perceive this personal investment in their work as either accidental or in conflict with an objective perspective on religion. Paradoxically, these writers insist that personal investment is what guarantees that their studies will not be distorted by "theology." It is only when persons remain open themselves to the gifting of "religion" that they will be able to resist the pressure to adhere to any one theology. Personal investment, in other words, provides people with a perspective—one that does not adhere too closely to the form of a religious phenomenon (theology in particular) and mire reason in the shape of the experience it represents, nor one that adheres too closely to methods (in opposition to theology) for translating the meaning of a phenomenon into rational terms. In either case, personal investment helps people refuse to surrender their reason to particular forms of its own reflections, or arrest the dynamic in which encounters with new phenomena serve to expand and correct their knowledge.

What the examples of Kant and Schleiermacher suggest is that every attempt to name a phenomenon as "religion" places a scholar in an ambiguous position vis-á-vis the phenomenon—somewhere between evangelism and disrespect. In so far as naming something "religion" involves offering a rational account of what cannot be rationally proven, "emergence" from "theology" is not an option. Nor is theology mere material to which scholars can apply their rational theories. Rather, in order to generate insights into religion—insights that adequately and critically represent what they claim to represent—scholars must maintain an engaged and self-conscious perspective on any claims to absolute knowledge, and do so through the practice of writing. In this respect, there is no ground outside a scholar's own relationship to religion on which to base a purely objective perspective. In questions of religion, such a position is impossible.

Proponents of an emergence narrative of the field who accuse Kant and Schleiermacher as insufficiently liberated from Christian theology are correct to a point; Kant and Schleiermacher embrace personal investment in religion as a condition for critical theory. Nevertheless, critics often fail to appreciate the ways in which efforts to move beyond these thinkers repeat what they criticize. Scholars in the contemporary study of religion remain rooted in the paradigm of knowledge evident in Kant and Schleiermacher. They take as given the capacity of reason to reflect upon the contents and processes of human experience, the limitations to knowledge imposed on reason by the contents and processes of experience, and the conviction that such writing-enabled reflection produces worthwhile knowledge. Thus, while seeking to resist the theological distortion they attribute to Kant and Schleiermacher, scholars follow the example of Kant and

Schleiermacher, hewing to practices of writing and models of language. The difference is that those who embrace an emergence narrative of the field refuse to accept the moments of affirmation and critique as comprising an irreducible paradox that is generative of the field. Instead they target the coexistence of the two moments as a sign of theological distortion and strive to reduce or resolve the tension to one side or the other. Yet, in doing so, critics appeal to a standard of objectivity that transcends the relationship between scholar and religion in which religion appears. Such a move, by their own account, is "theological"—it is a move that both Kant and Schleiermacher criticize. It is a move that presumes that writing is the practice that best trains reason to negotiate the rift between affirmation and critique animated in every use of the term "religion." There is no way to extricate personal investment from the project of studying religion without unraveling the epistemological paradigm within which the term "religion" occurs.

This analysis suggests that it may be helpful for the case of dance to read the history of the field differently—not as a story of emerging from theology, but as a story of an ongoing, generative tension between attempts to theorize religion, on the one hand, and conceptions and uses of theology, on the other. In the context of this narrative of generative tension, already suggested by my readings of Kant and Schleiermacher, it is possible to acknowledge the strategic role played by writing as a disciplinary practice in the study and ongoing life of religion. Such a perspective would encourage attention to how the practice of writing enables and angles our approach to religion, and thus open a similar register of questions we might pose, as I do in Part 2, to dance.

First, however, close readings of Hegel and Kierkegaard, in chapters 3 and 4 respectively, offer further resources for thinking through the relationship between writing and dancing that is presumed by attempts to study religion.

Doing the Work of Spirit
G. W. F. Hegel

The discussions in Chapters 1 and 2 map two conceptual axes that continue to define the terms of contemporary debates over "religion": one stretching between a core of religion and its phenomenal forms and a second, within that definition of core, stretching between rational belief and inner experience. Chapters 3 and 4 engage this terrain in ways that open a third dimension: that between "religion" (so defined by these two axes) and the scientific study of it. Georg Wilhelm Friedrich Hegel (1770-1831) articulates this distinction as a way to accomplish what he perceives Kant and Schleiermacher do not: to offer a theory of religion that is both affirming and critical. Kierkegaard contests Hegel's solution and evokes the image of *dancing* to figure what Hegel's "Science" of religion is incapable of comprehending. In setting up the opposition between dancing and philosophical writing, Kierkegaard's response to Hegel suggests that a particular kind of disregard for "dance" arises as an enabling correlate of the emergence narrative of the field.

LOSING RELIGION

Hegel's critiques of the theories of religion represented in this book by Kant and Schleiermacher drive the argument of his first great philosophical work, the *Phenomenology of Spirit* (1806).[1] After years as headmaster at the Gymnasium in Nurenberg, and then as a professor at the Universities of Heidelberg (1816-8) and Berlin (1818-1831), Hegel returned to flesh out the implications of his critiques, offering a series of lectures on the "philosophy of religion," which he gave in 1821, 1824, 1827, and 1831. Although Hegel never assembled these lectures for publication, scholars have pieced them together from his notes and those of students.[2] While the specifics of his analyses evolve over the ten-year period, his underlying critique is consistent: the theories of religion represented by the likes of Kant and Schleiermacher fail (with echoes of Schleiermacher) because they fail to *affirm* the *particularity* of the myriad historical manifestations of religion. The problem Hegel discerns is that such thinkers, in the rush to provide a *rational* defense of religion, yield the terms of the argument to those they seek to persuade. They predicate their theories on a *distinction* between reason and experience authorized by the successes of "science." Not only do they take this distinction as given, they also emphasize one side of the distinction as representing a *core* or concept of religion over and against the other that to them represents its external forms. For Hegel, it is in this sense that their theories are one-sided and "theological." They are "theological" in so far as neither approach is able to support as *positive* another human's claims to the absolute. Religious symbols, doctrines, or actions—including instances of dance—can appear only as arbitrary if imaginative elaborations of either a rational belief or an experience of sensory immersion. We have seen as much in the chapters above.

The examples Hegel gives demonstrate the stakes of his critique and gesture towards his response. On the one hand, Hegel insists that identifying the core of religion with rational belief in God breeds a nearly "universal indifference toward the doctrines of faith formerly regarded as essential" (LPR 82). Through such a lens, the "work of salvation" attributed to Jesus Christ by orthodox dogmatics, for example, assumes mere "psychological" significance (LPR 82). The same holds true for articles of faith, the Trinity, miracles, and eternal life. As Hegel observes, the situation is such that "the educated public" and "many theologians" would be "embarrassed to have to declare" themselves about such claims (LPR 83). In ceding the terms of the debate to scientific culture, such theories and theologies lose the ability to affirm the positive content of religious traditions.

On the other hand, Hegel insists, a philosophy of religion that locates the core of religion in an irreducible moment of experience fares no better in affirming the particular forms and content of religious life. While such an approach honors the capacity of humans to sense infinity, it does so by denying cognition an active role in religion: "The immediacy of the connectedness is taken as precluding the alternative determination of mediation . . . one knows *that* God is, *not what* God is. The expansion, the content, the fulfillment of the representation of God is thus negated" (LPR 87-8). When scholars take this dichotomy between immediate and mediate forms of knowledge as fixed and given, any attempts to make positive statements about God or establish ethical norms in relation to God again appear as "arbitrary" (LPR 93). Any intuition of the universe signifies negatively, as a sign of a desire for what is not and cannot be present.

For Hegel, then, a definition of religion's core predicated on a distinction between reason and experience fails to offer an adequate critique or affirmation of religion because religion itself appears as impossible. Either humans have immediate knowledge of a God they cannot comprehend, or they have mediated knowledge about a God they can never know. Summarizing the tension between the two positions, Hegel writes: "This polarization seems to be the Gordian knot with which scientific culture is at present struggling, and which it still does not properly understand. One side boasts of its wealth of materials and intelligibility, the other side at least scorns this intelligibility, and flaunts its immediate rationality and divinity" (PS §14, 8). It is a Gordian knot that structures the antitheology polemics of today as well, pitting those who advocate "intelligibility" via scientific

method against those who defend "divinity" via respect for difference, with each side accusing the other of being too "theological."
Hegel would agree: both sides are right.

A NEW SCIENCE

As a basis for a theory of religion capable of providing a critical affirmation of the particular shapes of religious life, Hegel proposes a new
Science—one that is not based on a simple *distinction* between reason
and experience. In response to those who would assert the privilege of
reason over experience or experience over reason (however defined),
Hegel embraces both vectors of influence as two moments in a *dialectical* rhythm. It is this rhythm between reason and experience, Hegel
avers, that gives rise to consciousness. It is a rhythm at work in any
concept of religion's core as well as in all phenomenal forms of religion in history. The name for this rhythm, Hegel writes, is "spirit."

In explaining the dialectic between reason and experience, Hegel
further elucidates what he means by "spirit." As Hegel explains, any
shape of consciousness is comprised of two moments: "knowing and
the objectivity negative to knowing," that is, a sense of an "I" who
knows and a sense of something known, whether object, person, concept, or truth (PS §36, 21). Consciousness is a relation. It is also
dynamic. When something appears to someone, in Hegel's language,
it does so by negating the subject; it appears as "not-I." Yet, as soon
as a distinction between "I" and "it" appears, consciousness recognizes both moments as internal to its own activity. The sense of "I"
expands, preserving and transcending these two moments in the
shape of a new "I." The "I" opens to a new "it," and the distinction
impels yet another act of sublating (*aufheben*), that is, negating, preserving, and transcending that distinction. In this dialectic, "experience" names the moment in which something appears to an "I" as
"alien" to itself, as something real and immediate and other breaking
in from elsewhere.[3] "Reason," in turn, names the moment in which a

person perceives this distinction between "I" and "it," between reason and experience as enabled by his own rational, sensory activity.[4] And "spirit" is the name for the movement that binds both movements in an irreducible interdepence. Nothing can appear to an "I" as immediately given (i.e., experience) unless that "I" already has the capacity of representing something to itself as not itself (i.e., can reason). Thus, reason enables experience, just as experience enables the coming into maturity of reason. The act of reason negates, preserves and transcends an experience; a new experience negates, preserves and transcends the previous self-understanding of reason. As Hegel writes, "Here we see pure consciousness posited in a twofold manner: once as the restless movement to and fro through all its moments, aware in them of an otherness which is superseded in the act of grasping it; and again, rather as the *tranquil unity* certain of its [own] truth," a "tranquil unity" that exists in and with and because of this restlessness (PS §237, 143). "Spirit," then, is the name Hegel chooses for this perception of consciousness as the dialectical movement (via reason and experience) of its own ongoing becoming.[5] The movement of spirit is never-ending.

What renders "spirit" most useful for the study of religion, however, is that it is not only a name for the dynamic at work in an individual consciousness. In so far as consciousness represents a relationship to truth, spirit is also a name for "the absolute," or "the true" itself. As Hegel writes: "The True is the whole . . . nothing other than the essence consummating itself through its development" (§20,11). As "the whole," the true is not a kind of thing that can be represented in the form of an idea or principle; it encompasses and includes *all*. In so far as it includes all, it must necessarily include the conditions of its own becoming, including the thinking, feeling, and sensing of individual human beings in their efforts to attain knowledge of the true. In other words, to see the true as "the whole" is to see that the true comes into being through a dialectical interplay of reason and experience. It is to see that the true is (the movement of) spirit.

For Hegel, then, the task of those who practice his Science is to learn to see spirit. Such philosophers must learn to see the dialectic of reason and experience not only in the rhythms of their own consciousness, but in every shape of life. The goal for Hegel is to be able to see history as a progression of shapes of consciousness, each arising necessarily from another. Philosophers who seek truth in the form of spirit endeavor to see every shape of human consciousness—including their own—as an (reason-enabled) *experience* for spirit; they perceive their own reflection on those shapes as the acts of (experience-enabled) *reason* through which spirit "knows itself." In sum, for Hegel, his "Science" marks the moment in history where human beings (as moments of spirit) come to see their own reasoning activity (in negating, preserving and transcending historical shapes of consciousness) as the activity of truth becoming—as spirit.[6] In Hegel's terms, "Spirit becomes object [in human consciousness] because it is just this movement of becoming an *other to itself*" (PS §36, 21; brackets mine).

SPIRIT IN RELIGION

Turning his concept of spirit to religion, Hegel offers a definition designed to negate, preserve, and transcend the distinction between reason and experience as assumed by earlier theorists. He describes "religion" as the thought *and* feeling of God:

> Everything that people value and esteem, everything on which they think to base their pride and glory, all of this finds its focal point in religion, in the thought or consciousness of God and the feeling of God. God is the beginning and end of all things. God is the sacred center, which animates and inspires all things . . . This concept of religion is universal. Religion holds this position for all peoples and persons. (LPR 76)

Whether or not "all peoples and persons" would agree with this concept of religion, Hegel's intention is to include; he aims to explain how thinking and feeling, or rational belief and inner experience, are both necessary and in fact comprise interlocking moments in the life of "religion." On the one hand, Hegel affirms with Kant and against Schleiermacher that "human beings think, and they alone have religion. From this it is to be concluded that religion has its inmost seat in thought" (LPR 121). In so far as religious consciousness presumes a relation of human beings to something absolute, then there can be no religion for a person who cannot elevate his thinking over and against the contents of sensory experience—"the sensible, the external, the singular"—and entertain an idea of something that transcends these particular sensory manifestations.7 Without the power of the thinking-I to negate sensory experience, there can be no *religious* consciousness.

On the other hand, with Schleiermacher and against Kant, Hegel contests that the object to which a person elevates her thinking gaze in religion "is also not an inert, abstract universal . . . but rather the absolute womb or the infinite fountainhead out of which everything emerges, in to which everything returns, and in which it is eternally maintained" (LPR 122)—a never-ending movement of positing and overcoming differences, or spirit.8 As a result, in order to know this absolute as the *Subject* that it is, and not just as *Substance*, thinking free from sensory experience is not enough: a person must also be able to (re)experience the sensible and particular as (manifestations of) this "absolute womb." She must be able to feel as true in and for herself the idea she can think.

Nor is it enough for Hegel that a person think and feel in relation to the absolute. He must understand how thinking and feeling give rise to one another and grasp their dialectical interdependence. As Hegel writes: "*The true* is their unity, *an immediate knowledge that likewise mediates*, a mediated knowledge that is at the same time internally simple, or is immediate reference to itself" (LPR 99). Hegel explains that unity does not imply dissolution: "the difference emphatically does not disappear, for it belongs to the pulse of its vitality, to the impetus, motion, and restlessness of spiritual as well as of natural life. Here is a unification in which the difference is not extinguished, but all the same it is sublated" (LPR 99). Any faith or feeling associated with religion is mediated by an ability to think an absolute; faith or feeling is "a wholly relative moment of origin" (LPR 141). Any idea of the absolute as Subject, in order to be true, must feel true for the person who thinks it. In short, there is no one thought or feeling in which the two dimensions of religion can coexist. A person's thinking and feeling of the absolute are "united" or sublated in a *rhythm* that constantly produces their difference. Said otherwise, the idea that religion is *spirit* implies that "religion" represents a person's ongoing movement, back and forth, between positing (in thought) and realizing (in feeling) a reconciliation—or knowledge—of him or herself with whatever he or she represents as "a sacred center."

In short, from the perspective of spirit, Kant's approach to religion is one-sided: he misses the influence of experience on the shape of rational belief. Schleiermacher's approach is also one-sided: he minimizes the influence of rational thinking on the shapes of religious experience. The choice they pose is a Gordian knot of intelligibility and divinity, and Hegel wants to secure both by reconceiving the relationship between reason and experience as a dialectical unity, spirit.

Even so, Hegel could be criticized as equally one-sided—that is, as privileging his concept of a thinking/feeling dialectic over and against the phenomenal forms of religious life—if he did not make an additional move. Hegel agrees: "Religion in its concept is not yet the true religion. The concept is true within itself, to be sure; but it also belongs to its truth that it should realize itself" (LPR 102). In so far as he, as a philosopher, can *think* about religion as a dialectical interplay of reason and experience, then he must also understand that his knowledge of religion is not complete. As a concept, the idea is abstract, "theoretical," and thus not what it claims to be. The concept of religion "still lacks the *practical* element, which comes to expression in the cultus" (LPR 189). Only in the "cultus"—that is, in the phenomenal forms of religion, the rituals, art, ethical actions, doctrines, community-building, etc.—does the *concept* of religion (as an interplay of thinking and feeling) realize the truth it represents. It becomes true for someone as the content of his or her relationship to the absolute. As Hegel writes, inhabiting the perspective of a religious consciousness,

> God is on one side, I am on the other, and the determination is *the including, within my own self, of myself with God,* the knowing of myself within God and of God within me. The cultus involves giving oneself this supreme, absolute enjoyment. There is feeling within it; I take part in it with my particular subjective personality, knowing myself as this individual included in and with God, knowing myself within the truth (and I have my truth only in God), i.e., joining myself as myself in God together with myself. (LPR 191)

Religion as an *idea* of reconciliation with the absolute, is false. It is only true in its "determinations," that is, in the particular forms of belief and practice through which an individual knows her particular self as reconciled with the absolute (LPR 191).

With this move, Hegel lays the groundwork for the field of religious studies: From here on, the task of defining a concept of religion must proceed hand in hand with careful attention to the actual historical forms of religion in the world. Philosophers of religion must, moreover, not do so as a way simply to test or challenge their hypotheses, but because the very concept of religion as spirit demands it. Scholars of religion must acknowledge that their rational reflections on religion are always already pulled and stretched by their experiences of historical religions—including their own. As a result, they must cultivate their experiences of religion as the context out of which their thinking about religion arises. Only by participating in this dialectic, Hegel's notion of cultus implies, will they be able to see spirit in the conceptual and phenomenal forms of religion.

Carrying this concept of a dialectical interplay between religion's concept (as itself a dialectial thinking and feeling of the absolute) and determinate forms (as the cultus) to its conclusion, Hegel rests his case. By learning to see spirit, a philosopher can generate a theory of religion that provides criteria for both identifying religious phenomena in their particularity, and acknowledging all forms as necessary moments in the life of spirit—that is, as "rational." As Hegel confirms, "The main point is to know that these appearances, wild as they are, are rational—to know that they have their ground in reason, and to know what sort of reason is in them" (LPR 430-1), whether theoretical or practical. Hegel's "main point" implies that a philosopher of religion must begin with the assumption that all historical religious phenomena are rational in so far as they are moments in the life of spirit. They represent someone's rational reflection on experience. Thus, discerning how these phenomena are "rational" does not imply holding phenomena to a pre-existing standard. Instead, a philosopher must allow his experience of the phenomena to inform his sense of what reason is and of how spirit works in the world. Hegel's intention here, though we may argue with the results, is to provide a ground for including, honoring, and affirming the myriad expressions of religious life in their particularity, as relevant for what I can think and know as true about religion.

As Hegel admits, the task of seeing spirit in the forms of religious life is not without danger. It can be difficult to discern what sort of reason a given form of religion represents.[9] Yet, in so far as she can recognize even the strangest of twists, a philosopher *saves* religion from one-sided theological approaches that would eviscerate religion by ceding the terms of its defense to scientific culture. Thus, Hegel concludes, it is the philosopher as opposed to the "theologian" who can "deal with religion more impartially on the one hand, and more fruitfully and auspiciously on the other" (LPR 79).

DOING THE WORK OF SPIRIT

However, as any attention to Hegel's discussion of the historical shapes of religion attests, it is not clear that the process of seeing a given shape as a moment in spirit does do justice to its particularity. All historical forms appear as stages enroute to the form of religion in which the relationship between human and the absolute is represented as "consummated," namely (Protestant) Christianity. What, then, guarantees that Hegel's Science of religion—as dynamic and historically sensitive as he intends it to be—adequately represents the phenomena that he recognizes by the name of religion? How does Hegel avoid the critique (again) that he levels against earlier "theologians": that they privilege a rationally defensible concept of religion (no matter how dialectically sophisticated) over and above its phenomenal forms?

Hegel has a response and, not surprisingly, it is spirit. Moving with his argument for now will lead us farther along the path to understanding the implications of his work for attending to dance as religion. For Hegel, a person who can think about truth as spirit and who can recognize the conceptual and phenomenal forms of "religion" as spirit, will come to understand that his reflections on religion are also moments in the dynamic self-manifestation that spirit is. In other words, a scholar realizes that his reflections on the concept of religion and on the determinate forms of religions share a logic, a goal, and a history with what he studies. Moreover, what they share is participation in a dialectical interplay that gives rise to each and to their relations. For Hegel, it is this common participation by religion and the Science of it in the life of spirit that guarantees that the philosopher's insights are both adequate to the phenomenon at hand and sufficiently objective.

How Hegel arrives at this conclusion sheds light on the significance that philosophical writing has for him—a significance that aligns his work with the theorists considered above who position themselves against dance. First, in so far as religion and the Science of it both participate in spirit, philosophers are guaranteed a degree of empathy with any form of religion as it informs their reflections on it. As Hegel asserts repeatedly, philosophy and religion share the same object: "our relation to God" (LPR 196). Both human activities are directed not only towards comprehending the human relation to the absolute, but also towards bringing human and absolute together in a form of knowledge—what Hegel calls "Absolute Knowing," in which humans know the Absolute and know themselves as the Absolute knowing itself. The difference, then, between religion and the Science of it for Hegel lies not in content or goal, but in form. In religion, the human thinking and feeling about God that is manifest in its phenomenal forms appears in figurative guise—as *representations*. In philosophy, that same content appears in conceptual form— as the notion of spirit. This common participation in spirit, then, acts as a brake on what philosophers see. They are looking to see what it is about a given phenomenon that enables them to think about it at all. They are not just looking to see reflections of themselves per se, but rather to see a logic of becoming similar to that which animates their own dialectic of reason and experience.

A second implication follows. Where common participation in spirit allows a degree of empathy, the difference Hegel notes between figurative and conceptual form implies a relationship between philosophy and religion that has a dialectical character. Hegel confirms this character in several ways, arguing that philosophy sublates religion in general, and theology in particular. In his *Lectures* he writes: "The first relationship that we considered was that of knowledge, the theoretical relationship [i.e., the concept of religion]. The second is the practical relationship or the knowledge of this elevation [i.e., the determinate forms of historical religions] . . . . The third moment is the knowing of this knowing. That is actual religion" (LPR 197; brackets mine). "The knowing of this knowing" is *implicit* for Hegel in the Christian picture of God who becomes human; it is *explicit* in the philosophical concept of spirit. The Science of religion is thus "actual religion" in so far as it actualizes religion: it negates the figurative form of religion, preserves its content (the reconciled relation of human and absolute), and transcends the particular form of that representation by offering a vision of world history, and not just of one tradition, as spirit.

For those who are concerned with affirming the particular forms of religious life (as Hegel himself claims to be), this idea of philosophy as "actual religion" is troubling. It suggests that the Science of religion will explain away religion; that we should all become philosophers. The balance seems tipped far too far to the side of critique. Even though Hegel admits that without the historical forms of religion it would not have become possible to think the concept of spirit, and even though he insists that people interested in religion must allow the concrete instances of history to push and pull their thinking into new forms of understanding "religion," the assumption of a dialectical relationship implies that philosophy can do religion better than religion can itself.

In a rhythm we have come to expect, Hegel checks this possibility, at least in part. He insists that this idea of philosophy as "actual religion" is itself abstract and false unless and until a philosopher can experience her own philosophizing activity—her thinking and writing—as the work of spirit in the world. Philosophy is not just an idea about religion (as thinking and feeling, concept and form); it is not just a rational theory about religion. Science of religion, for Hegel, is a phenomenal form *of religion* appearing in history. As Hegel avers: "philosophy [too] is a continual cultus." He elaborates: "it has as its object the true, and the true in its highest shape as absolute spirit, as God. To know this true not only in its simple form as God, but also to know the rational in God's works—as produced by God and endowed with reason—that is philosophy" (LPR 194). Here, Hegel's designation of philosophy as cultus continues his critique of one-sided, theological approaches to the study of religion. Scholars of religion cannot rest in an abstract theory of religion. In so far as they seek the truth of religion, they participate in what religion itself represents—a human relation to the true. Only by acknowledging this common participation in a dialectic of reason and experience will philosophers be able to appreciate the differences in form.

In likening philosophy to a "continual cultus," Hegel places an additional check on the possibility that a philosopher will project abstract theories onto religious phenomena. To know the "rational in God's works," he explains, requires discipline—a practice of engaging in a dialectical interplay of reason and experience. Hegel continues: "It is part of knowing the true that one should dismiss one's subjectivity, the subjective fancies of personal vanity, and concern oneself with the true purely in thought, conducting oneself solely in accordance with objective thought. This negation of one's specific subjectivity is an essential and necessary moment" (LPR 194-5). On the one hand, negating one's "specific subjectivity" is a precondition of all thinking. As Hegel holds, reason develops its freedom over and against the finite forms of past experience. At the same time, however, a philosopher must engage in this self-dismissal when encountering the historical forms of religion. In other words, he must dismiss his subjective fancies and allow his consciousness to be pulled and stretched by the "pure thought" present in what appears to him.[10]

For Hegel, such a dismissing of subjectivity is not accidental to the process of understanding spirit. It is the crucial moment. If a philosopher does not negate her subjectivity, she cannot grasp her relation to the material at hand as spirit. Only when she sets aside her subjective fancies will she be able to see what she shares with what initially appears as very different, namely participation in this logic of becoming through a process of surrendering to experience. Thus, in so far as a philosopher practices dismissing her subjectivity, she comes to know herself, paradoxically, as enacting the reconciliation that Hegel's concept of religion promises. Philosophy, in this sense, is "actual religion." A philosopher works actively to acknowledge all other persons, regardless of sex, class, nationality, or creed, as participating in the life of spirit. As Hegel confirms, "If heart and will are earnestly and thoroughly cultivated for the universal and the true, then there is present what appears as *ethical life*. To that extent ethical life is the most genuine cultus" (LPR 194). The practice of philosophy is "actual religion" in so far as it implies an attitude of love towards all persons, not just those in one's particular tradition.[11]

Finally, as Hegel insists, the rhythm of dismissing "subjective fancies" and coming to know oneself (in relation to a new phenomenon) as spirit is "continual." There is no end to the process. There is no end to the manifestations of spirit in relation to which a person must negate himself and the difference of that manifestation from himself. In these ways, then, Hegel seeks to affirm the myriad forms of religious life—from ideas to practices, Hindu to Christian—in their *particularity* as *rational* in so far as they guide humans to perceive their responsibility for realizing ethical community.[12]

In sum, Hegel's reading of religion has implications for the relation of religious studies to theology that the emergence narrative of the field fails to grasp. In so far as "theology" represents one of religion's phenomenal forms, the implication is that a philosopher of religion depends upon theology not only for material to study, but also as a check to his "subjective fancies." The forms of theology exert pressure on reason; reason must stretch itself to identify with them and learn about spirit from them. Said otherwise, the ability of a philosopher to launch a critical affirmation of religion depends upon a dialectical engagement with theology. As Hegel insists: "The result of the study of philosophy is that those walls of division [between philosophy and theology], which are supposed to separate absolutely, become transparent" (LPR 91). Hegel's point is not that the walls disappear. A difference remains. Yet whatever arises as "theology" and whatever arises as "philosophy of religion" should do so in full view of the other. This transparency, Hegel implies, is essential for the efficacy of each discipline: for theology in which figurative representations are crafted through which people can come to know themselves as reconciled with God, and for philosophy, in which some people, at least, can work to realize those principles of reconciliation on a world stage.

Hegel may not have traveled along this path towards historical phenomena far enough to please contemporary critics. His notion of spirit seems too unscientific. A Christian-informed idea of reason still seems to prevail. The historical forms he describes appear as caricatures. At the same time, Hegel discerns what scholars in the field are only beginning to acknowledge: that the attempt to distance a scientific study of religion from "theology" actually undermines the objective quality of that science. As Hegel explains, what allows a philosopher to do justice to both the concept and the phenomenal forms of "religion" is a consciousness of how his study participates in the life of what "religion" represents to him. He writes: "Religion exists only in self-consciousness; outside that it exists nowhere" (LPR 160). The point here is not that "religion" is a figment of a scholar's imagination, but that a Science of religion entails a constant, ongoing interrogation of what "religion" means in and through a process of (re)experiencing historical phenomena: As we shall see, van der Leeuw picks up and amplifies this aspect of Hegel's work.

WRITING PHILOSOPHY

Despite all of the ways in which Hegel's Science of religion advances positions represented by Schleiermacher and Kant, in the end he shares with them a strategy for negotiating the moments of critique and affirmation that enforces a tendency to discount dancing as making a positive contribution to religious meaning. Where *philosophy* is a continual cultus, the medium in and through which the performance of that cultus occurs—the medium through which the concept of spirit becomes actual—is *writing*. Here Hegel's Science falls in line: he relies on the practice of writing to enact the relationship between reason and experience on which he constructs his theory of religion. It is the act of writing that provides philosophers with the experience in and through which they come to understand their scholarly activity as the work of spirit in the world.

For one, writing is the act a philosopher performs in order to exercise his powers of rational thinking in *overcoming* the distinction between his sense of himself as a reasoner and the forms of religion that impress him. In order to study religion, Hegel counsels, it is not necessary for a philosopher to experience all forms of religion for himself. Rather, he must read and write about them, "devouring" these experiences as his "inorganic nature" (PS §28, 16). In reading, he allows historical phenomena to confront him, to negate him. As such, it is in the process of reading and writing that he becomes conscious of the movement of consciousness or spirit that binds his reason with the forms of experience he studies.

At the same time, Hegel acknowledges that writing is not only a mental activity. It is cultus, an embodied action. As such, writing expresses a philosopher's specific subjectivity. *She* sits, thinks, writes. As such, the same activity through which a philosopher exercises her ability to find the rational in experience and deny her subjective personality also exercises and expresses her individuality. Moreover, it expresses and enhances that individuality by helping a person realize her embodied thinking and writing as the action of spirit coming to know itself. By writing philosophically about religion, she is and knows herself as the movement of *Aufhebung*. The act of writing provides her with an experience of herself as making real for herself her *own* reconciliation with what religion represents.

In this way the practice of writing performs a function for Hegel similar to the function it performed for Kant and Schleiermacher: it serves to space the relationships between reason and experience, and scholar and religion, so as to strike a desirable combination of affirmation and critique. For Hegel's philosopher, writing works both directly and indirectly. On the one hand, writing exercises and strengthens a philosopher's ability to wield the concept of spirit in analyzing and disclosing the rational content of religion. On the other, writing also enacts his empathetic connection with religion, in so far as the writer appreciates his own writing about religion as "actual religion," as religion realizing its truth. Philosophical writing thus enacts the reconciliation of human and spirit, of religion and the Science of religion. Philosophical writing reveals the truth of religion by being the truth of religion.

Hegel summarizes his view:

> In so far as thinking begins to posit an antithesis to the concrete and places itself in opposition to the concrete, the process of thinking consists in carrying through this opposition until it arrives at reconciliation. This reconciliation is philosophy. Philosophy is to this extent theology. It presents the reconciliation of God with himself and with nature, showing that nature, otherness, is implicitly divine, and that the raising of itself to reconciliation is on the one hand what finite spirit implicitly is [as the experience of Spirit], while on the other hand it arrives at this reconciliation, or brings it forth, in world history. This reconciliation is the peace of God, which does not "surpass all reason," but is rather the peace that *through* reason is first known and thought and is recognized as what is true. (LPR 489; my brackets)

At first glance, this passage provides much fodder for an antitheology polemic. Hegel admits that his Science of religion is "to this extent" theology. However, Hegel is also making the point that philosophy cannot offer a rational critical account of religion unless it engages theology in a dialectical way through the practice of writing. The very gesture involved in reaching to acknowledge a phenomenon as "religion" implies an ethic. It implies the possibility of understanding, the existence of some kind of connection, and a desire for bringing self and object of study into a new relationship. It is on this ground that Hegel argues that a philosopher writing about religion is always already part and parcel of what he studies. As Hegel writes: "In intuition or the theoretical relationship there is only one object with which I am filled; I know nothing of myself. The true, however, is the relationship of myself and this object" (LPR 190). Hegel's challenge to us is to admit that "to this extent," though not entirely, any attempt to study religion may indeed be theology, presenting and realizing a reconciliation of myself and this object.

DANCING SPIRIT

Hegel's Science is inherently dynamic and alive. Spirit is a vision of truth *as* movement: truth is not some entity that moves, it is (itself) moving. Though we may think about "spirit" as if it were a substance, Hegel insists that any ideas humans can conceive, no matter how kinetic, are false. To know spirit as movement is to know spirit in and as the activity of my own thinking, feeling, sensing, desiring, and writing. To know spirit is to know the human relation to truth as a dynamic process in which both human beings and their conceptions of truth evolve in relation to one another, over time and through space. A human is truth-becoming.

Critics who decry Hegel as an "archrationalist" (ready to consign women and others to the "all conquering force of reason in history"), or as an "idealist" (for whom the idea of spirit determines all reality), assume that Hegel's "Absolute Knowing" is static in form and content.[13] The reading above suggests a different interpretation. Where spirit is the dialectical interplay of reason and experience, and philosophy a "continual cultus," it follows that the unity of that dialectic cannot occur within the realm of "reason" over and against the realm of "experience." As Hegel makes clear in his *Lectures*, when a person uses reason to discern spirit in the historical and phenomenological forms of religion, what she can think about religion cannot be true unless her rational knowing can be sublated in an action (namely writing) that allows her to feel as true for her embodied existence the idea of religion she can think. In this respect, any "unity" of reason and experience consists of a rhythm—a logic of bodily becoming—in which the two are interdependent moments. As an idea, then, Absolute Knowing is a call to act in ways that realize ethical communities.

Because Hegel endorses this dialectical relation between reason and experience, his theory of religion moves further towards dance than the positions described in earlier chapters. Here, it seems, there might be room for affirming dance as a practice that allows a person to experience his own bodily movement as spirit moving in and as and through him. At the same time, Hegel's identification of *philosophy* as cultus narrows that possibility in so far as the model and form for philosophical activity is writing. For Hegel, it is in and through the process of writing about spirit that a person comes to know his own relation with spirit. Although Hegel admits that writing can serve this function because it is a concrete, embodied activity, he still seems to suggest that writing works by translating a person's particular subjectivity into rational forms. Writing individualizes and embodies *reason* in its ability to overcome the distinction between reason and experience. In writing, a person proves for himself the truth of values, norms, and concepts that are publicly available.

Thus, where writing emerges as an activity uniquely suited to sustaining a dialectical tension between reason and experience—that is, where writing emerges as sign and medium for realizing a dialectical unity of human and the Absolute, finite and infinite—then the balance Hegel intends to strike between reason and experience falls to the side of reason. Even though philosophical writing expresses an individual's will-in-action, the *telos* of that experience remains a knowledge of myself-with-God which can be shared with a reading public through the writing process.

It is at this point that Hegel falls prey to the critiques often leveled against his Science. Once a philosopher learns to *write* about spirit as spirit, why bother with religion at all?

CHAPTER 4

The Poet and the Dancer

Søren Kierkegaard

In several of his pseudonymous works, Søren Kierkegaard introduces dance as a figure for representing that aspect of religion that a Hegelian philosopher cannot comprehend: faith.[1] In these appearances, the metaphoric weight of the image does not depend on an opposition of the bodily to the intellectual, the outer to the inner, or the emotional to the rational. Dancing appears as religion. It appears as a way of inhabiting religion; it engages thinking, feeling, and enacting. Rather, in Kierkegaard's work, "dancing" has meaning as a kind of doing that eludes the grasp of philosophical writing. As this chapter reveals, by hinging his critique of Hegel's Science of religion on a difference between writing and dancing, Kierkegaard encapsulates both the difficulty and the potential value of developing theories and methods of religion capable of acknowledging dance as a medium of religious expression and experience.

In exploring these issues, this chapter offers a close reading of one of Kierkegaard's most beloved works: *Fear and Trembling* (1843). Kierkegaard in the guise of Johannes Silentio criticizes Hegel's Science for failing to explain how people *enter* his system, how they make the leap to believe in spirit and commit themselves to writing (as) "spirit."[2] As Silentio writes: "Even if someone were able to transpose the whole content of faith into conceptual form, it does not follow that he has comprehended faith, comprehended how he entered into it or how it entered into him."[3] The example Silentio gives of someone whom Hegel's philosophical writing cannot comprehend is Abraham. Abraham has faith. And by describing him as a dancer, Silentio foregrounds the relationship of writing to dancing as *a*, if not *the* crucial issue in the study of religion (and dance).

THE POET

Unlike the writers we have read in Chapters 1 through 3, Johannes Silentio is impelled to write about "religion" by a feeling of bafflement. He does not write in order to exercise his reason, nor piece together the shards of a fleeting experience, nor do the reconciling work of spirit. He writes from the point of view of someone who claims to understand and even admire Hegel's system for the extensive reach of its dialectical gaze. What he cannot understand, however, is how to see spirit—the dialectical rhythm of reason and experience—in the biblical account of Abraham and Isaac. When he attempts to translate Abraham's actions into conceptual forms, he is "paralyzed" (33). He cannot move. Abraham's willingness to sacrifice his son Isaac for God appears absurd and it is this lack of understanding that impels Silentio to write. He writes to trace the chasm between what Hegel claims concerning the power of philosophical writing, on the one hand, and the case of Abraham, on the other. He writes to make intelligible Abraham's unintelligibility, and to do so from several perspectives.[4] What Hegel's Science cannot grasp, Silentio suspects, is what sets spirit in motion. Describing his age, he laments that "not a word is heard about faith. Who speaks to the honor of this passion? Philosophy goes further. Theology sits all rouged and powdered in the window and courts its favor, offers its charms to philosophy. It is supposed to be difficult to understand Hegel, but to understand Abraham is a small matter" (32).[5]

As he is impelled by bafflement, Silentio further claims to have no interest in writing for a reading public. He writes for himself. As he avers, in an age "that has crossed out passion in order to serve science" (7), the reading public has developed a taste for a certain kind of writing—an expectation he does not intend to fulfill. As he insists: "The present author is by no means a philosopher... He writes because to him it is a luxury that is all the more pleasant and apparent the fewer there are who buy and read what he writes" (7). Not only does Silentio not write in order to know, he claims that he does not write to communicate to others what he knows. He writes rather more like a poet, to "admire, love and delight" in Abraham as a paradigm of faith. He is "recollection's genius" (15). By taking on the role of Silentio in relation to Abraham, then, Kierkegaard enacts the predicament of someone keen to write about religion. Silentio is someone whose expertise in philosophical writing enables him to appreciate faith as something that he cannot understand. Through Silentio, Kierkegaard raises questions about how education in the practice of writing opens and forecloses a particular relation to religion.

A "PRODIGIOUS PARADOX"

In his description of Abraham's faith, Silentio traces the outlines of a double movement he claims Hegel's Science cannot explain. In Abraham's story, what most puzzles Silentio is Abraham's *willingness*: how was Abraham willing to sacrifice his long-awaited only son, Isaac, to God—a son promised to him by God—without hating either God or Isaac? In an attempt to make sense of this willingness, Silentio traces two movements he thinks that Abraham must have made. The first is a movement of infinite resignation, something Silentio insists is easy enough to understand and replicate. In this movement, a person exercises her power to concentrate the "whole substance" of her life and love into a single desire, and concentrate the conclusion of her thinking into "one act of consciousness" (43). She chooses to renounce this "whole substance" in the name of a higher eternal and absolute Good as defining the source and telos of her particular existence. As Silentio describes, this resigning of self to the infinite is a "purely philosophical movement that I venture to make when it is demanded and can discipline myself to make, because every time some finitude will take power over me, I starve myself into submission until I make the movement, for my eternal consciousness is my love for God, and for me that is the highest of all" (48). This movement of resignation is thus akin to Hegel's movement of negation, the dismissing of subjective fancies, in which a thinking-I denies any determinative weight to the particulars of human life, including the contents of its own hopes and desires. For Hegel, as for Silentio, this philosophical move is a pre-condition for religion (and the study of it). A knight of infinite resignation transforms her desire for this life into an eternal longing for an absolute Other. Transcending the vicissitudes of worldly concern and pleasure, she finds peace and consolation from the tumult of desire. She knows that God's will will prevail. As Silentio surmises, Abraham must have made such a movement of infinite resignation—he loved God above all else. He loved God so much that he was willing to sacrifice Isaac, the whole substance of his life, for God, the "highest of all."

Nevertheless, Silentio contends, this move of infinite resignation does not explain Abraham's *willingness* to sacrifice Isaac. It does not explain, for one, how Abraham was able to *love* a God who would demand such act. God's request contradicts the idea of God as eternal love that inspires the move of infinite resignation. From the point of view of the infinite good, the act God demands of Abraham is unethical: "The ethical expression for what Abraham did is that he meant to murder Isaac; the religious expression is that he meant to sacrifice Isaac—but precisely in this contradiction is the anxiety that can make a person sleepless, and yet without this anxiety Abraham is not who he is" (30). Herein lies the horror that Hegel's Science cannot digest: even if Abraham were absolutely sure that the call to transgress his ethical obligation as a father came from God, how could he continue to love and trust a God who could contradict God's own nature? Such a love finds no ground or justification in any universal concept or norm; nor can consciousness stretch to reconcile such an experience in a dialectical unity. From a speculative point of view, such love is absurd.

Further, neither does the movement of infinite resignation explain how Abraham was able to persevere in loving Isaac once called upon to sacrifice him. It is one thing for Abraham to resign himself to losing Isaac; it is another to be willing to kill Isaac with his own hand. How could Abraham perform this deed as an expression of love? Again, from the point of view of Hegel's spirit, such love is irrational and dangerous.

Thus, what Silentio finds when he tries to see spirit in Abraham's faith is not a knowledge-generating dialectic of reason and experience, but an irreducible paradox. Abraham loves God; Abraham loves Isaac; the satisfactions demanded by these two loves cannot be reconciled. Moreover, there is no higher unity capable of preserving and transcending both loves: one of them and not just their apparent opposition must be negated. How then was Abraham able to justify his *willingness* to act? Why did he not shrink away in horror? Silentio intones: he had faith. Faith is what enabled Abraham to hold together these irreconcilable loves for the finite and the infinite.

Faith, Silentio concludes, involves a second movement beyond infinite resignation—a leap—where a person decides to believe that a God who is Absolute and infinite nonetheless cares about his finite, embodied well-being. In order to keep loving God *and* Isaac while agreeing to kill Isaac for God, Abraham must have believed that God would give him Isaac back, that God's self-contradiction was somehow not a contradiction. If Abraham cannot make this movement, Silentio contends, he relinquishes one of his loves and either resigns himself to God and renounces his love for Isaac, or affirms his love for Isaac and hates God for demanding such a sacrifice.

Yet Silentio protests: such a belief is absurd! For Abraham to believe in such a reconciliation and proceed with the sacrifice would be to place himself above the ethical commands that apply to all humans. How dare he? Silentio marvels that Abraham must have mustered some will to believe on no other grounds with no other incentive or insurance than that provided by the strength of his own dueling passions—his passion for God as absolute infinite goodness, and his passion for his son as the embodiment and whole substance of his life. In his passion, Abraham refuses to relinquish either of these conflicting loves; he holds together his love for the universal and for the particular, for the eternal and for the finite. Silentio concludes that Abraham has faith by virtue of the absurd. In Abraham's willingness to act, he never betrays his love for God or for Isaac, and for this reason, when God provides him with a ram for the sacrifice and an angel stays the hand he poises for the kill, Abraham is able to demonstrate the mental and emotional agility needed to embrace Isaac with joy and praise God. Silentio muses: "And yet what did he achieve? He remained true to his love. But anyone who loves God needs no tears, no admiration; he forgets the suffering in the love. Indeed, so completely has he forgotten it that there would not be the slightest trace of his suffering left if God himself did not remember it, for he sees in secret and recognizes distress and counts the tears and forgets nothing" (120). Abraham's own passion is his salvation.

THE DANCER

In writing about Abraham, Silentio admits that he cannot hope to communicate in rational terms Abraham's willingness to act. He writes instead in order to call his readers to admire, love, and delight in what he calls Abraham's leap—his dance. Describing the knight of faith, Silentio writes:

> He is continually making the movement of infinity, but he does it with such precision and assurance that he continually gets finitude out of it, and no one ever suspects anything else. It is

supposed to be the most difficult feat for a ballet dancer to leap into a specific posture in such a way that he never once strains for the posture but in the very leap assumes the posture. Perhaps there is no ballet dancer who can do it—but this knight does it. (40-1)

In Silentio's rendering, a knight of faith is moment by moment detaching himself (via the powers of philosophical thinking) from desired shapes of sensory experience; finding solace for his deprivation in concepts of an infinite absolute, and simultaneously, embracing the finite, temporal world, believing that he will receive, "totally and completely" the object of his desire (47-8). The postures through which the knight of faith moves are in this sense internal—rational, emotional, and existential. Why then liken the knight to a dancer—and a ballet dancer at that?[6]

As elsewhere in the text, in this passage the weight of Silentio's dance metaphor lies in a comparison with philosophical writing. "Dancing" enacts a different dialectical relation of reason and experience than that enacted by philosophical writing—a dialectic whose unity finds expression in a singular leap rather than a system.

To begin, part of the rhetorical power of the dance image rests with the style of dancing that Silentio mentions. Ballet in Copenhagen at the time was a polished and refined art, presided over by strict dancing masters who drilled dancers to develop technical prowess. The plots often figured supernatural themes, and the goal of the dancers, female and male, was to present an illusion of lightness and ease while executing complicated, technical feats.[7] Like the ballet dancers of Kierkegaard's day, Abraham projects an illusion of effortlessness in accomplishing movements that are extremely difficult to master.

What Abraham does that resembles the actions of a ballet dancer is to leap. The shape of a leap is also significant. A leap is a movement in which a dancer springs off the ground with one foot, hovers for a moment off the ground, and then lands on the other foot. As such, it embodies in one explosive action a double movement—a movement of leaving the earth and returning to it, like the knight of faith.[8] In a leap, as in faith, although the two movements contradict one another (going up, going down), they appear in that act as one seamless arc, connecting earth to earth. Yet this unity is not the unity of the system—it is not a unity gathered into a rational reflection by writing. The unity exists in the form of a singular, temporal, finite act. It exists only in passing—in the flash of its occurrence. As Silentio affirms: "Temporality, finitude—that is what it is all about" (49). The sole traces it leaves behind are buried within the kinetic awareness of the dancer, or the visual, visceral memory of the poet.

Moreover, Abraham's faith is like dancing rather than writing in the effort required. The process of passing through the various moments of a leap requires transformation. A dancer must *enter* a different "posture" or position. She must become a different shape in time and space; she lands on a different foot. As the movement is hers, this transformation is irreducibly subjective and individual. No one else can perform it for her. A dancer is not a puppet. To make the movement she cannot *not* coordinate her physical and mental energies, and focus them on the task at hand. Having faith, like leaping, expresses a concentration of an individual; it concentrates and individualizes an individual. It is through a faith like dance, Silentio insists, that a person becomes who she is: she exercises the relationship between reason and experience that defines her being in the world. She is not writing to exercise her reason for a reading public.

In addition, having faith, like making a leap, not only enacts the unity of two contradictory moments in a way that expresses individuality, it also reveals *by concealing* the network of conditions that make that movement possible. What the spontaneous explosion of a ballet leap both reveals and conceals are the years of training and practice required to develop the sense of timing, coordination, and physical consciousness necessary to perform successfully the action. Likewise, Abraham's willingness reveals and conceals—and reveals by concealing—the discipline and practice he must have in order to have faith. The knight of infinite resignation shows the strain. He can will himself up into the air with ease but stumbles when he lands. On the other hand, Abraham's calm demeanor masks the difficulty (from Silentio's point of view) of moving between an act of surrendering everything to God's will, and an act of believing that one's wishes will be met. Where a dancer's perfect landing incarnates grace, Abraham's joy at receiving Isaac incarnates infinite love in the finite shape of his body. For Silentio, it is dancing, not writing, that enacts the alchemy that faith requires: a knight of faith can "change the leap of life into walking, absolutely to express the sublime in the pedestrian" (41).

In sum, Silentio draws a contrast between dancing and writing that hinges on the intention, effort, process, and outcome of the two endeavors. While a philosopher writes to produce a system—an all-encompassing picture of what eternally is—Abraham's arduous dance training produces a leap. Where a philosopher writes to deliver himself from temporality and finitude—or at least, to affirm their dialectical unity with rational thinking—Silentio's knight enters temporality and finitude as the condition of his faith. In short, in Silentio's portrayal, Abraham's dancing exercises the dialectic of reason and experience by individualizing and embodying experience. Abraham, like Silentio, has made the move of infinite resignation—he can reason over and against his sensory experience and its various representations. Yet Abraham's dancing represents another movement as well—a move made after reason, beyond reason and writing, and into a different kind of experience: *passion*. What lies beyond a trained reason is a possibility for gathering and releasing a surge of energy and intention that an instant of dancing is. Abraham's leap is not a once-and-for-all movement that enables a person to find secure footing. A leaper lands on one foot, ready to leap, or walk, again. As such, faith is not something a person has; it is something he is endlessly doing.

By likening faith to dance in this way, Kierkegaard's Silentio not only provides insights into faith, but he also sheds additional light on why the philosophers described above tend to overlook dance in their attempts to theorize and study religion. From a point of view trained to detach "reason" from "experience," dancing looks like faith. Dancing appears to be a simple, nonverbal, pre-literate, unreflective incidence of sensory experience whose rational content human reason may translate, refine, and represent as knowledge in writing. Yet as Kierkegaard's use of Silentio suggests, this perception of dance as nonverbal is a function of a thinking mind disciplined by writing to believe in writing. As I discuss in more detail below, Silentio can see (Abraham) dancing only because he has had *and lost* faith in writing. For Kierkegaard, dancing proves a potent image for a critique of Hegel precisely because it has appeared to philosophers and theologians as marginal to the task of theorizing religion. It not only provides Kierkegaard with a figure for representing what Hegel's Science has failed to include, it helps him identify forces—namely the role of philosophical writing—that orchestrate and justify that exclusion.

Following this line of argument, Silentio's words about faith suggest a positive direction for theorizing dance as religion that van der Leeuw later develops. When Silentio claims that "faith is not the first immediacy, but a later immediacy" (82), he could be speaking for dance as well; it is not a first immediacy (i.e., natural movement), but a later one (i.e., movement that looks natural thanks to years of coordinated dedication of mental, emotional, and physical energies). Correlatively, Silentio's claim that faith "is not the spontaneous inclination of the heart but the paradox of existence" finds its echo in a theory of dance as enacting this paradox of existence, what van der Leeuw develops as a paradox of expression (47). As Silentio himself assures, to take part in this paradox—to cultivate the contradictory movements represented by love for God and love for world *as* the source of joy and love—is to "dance." "Most people," he notes, "live completely absorbed in the worldly joys and sorrows; they are bench-warmers who do not take part in the dance" (41).

Thus, in the culminating moment of faith to which Silentio acts as witness, the moments of rational reflection and sensory experience *are* reconciled in a dialectical unity, as they are for Hegel. That unity in Kierkegaard's work, though, appears in the form of a living, breathing, singular, embodied individual, not a system. It is a unity held together only in passion, not mere feeling, but the explosive concentration needed to fuse two contradictory movements into a complex and difficult leap.

DANCING CULTUS

As the parallels between dance and faith emerge in Silentio's writing about Abraham, so too does the heart of Kierkegaard's critique of Hegel: the very devotion to writing that causes Silentio to notice Abraham in the first place as an anomaly in need of explanation, is what, in the end, prevents him from understanding Abraham.[9] The same may be true for one who studies "religion."

Silentio notices Abraham because Silentio is a writer. He has made the movement of infinite resignation by appropriating the means if not the ends of Hegel's philosophy of religion. He has mastered the art of speculative reason; he can detach his thinking capacity from the contents and conditions of his experience, overcome the difference they represent, and express his reconciliation with those contents and conditions in writing. He delights in the power of his reasoning, writing "I" to negate the determining influences of doctrines or desires and conceive of an eternal absolute; he proclaims his love for an infinite "God," his commitment to ethics, and to the expression of rational knowledge. The fact that Silentio identifies himself as a writer is a sign that he has made the movement of infinite resignation.

At the same time, the degree to which Silentio holds to writing as the philosophical practice through which the peace of his resignation to the infinite is delivered is also the degree to which Abraham's faith provokes his anxiety. Even though he has mastered Hegel's system, Silentio cannot find the rational in Abraham's experience; he cannot reconcile Abraham to himself through his writing. He cannot make the movement of faith, nor convince himself that by writing about Abraham he is making it. As Silentio confesses:

> I cannot make the movement of faith, I cannot shut my eyes and plunge confidently into the absurd; it is for me an impossibility, but I do not praise myself for that. I am convinced that God is love. . . . To me God's love, in both the direct and converse sense, is incommensurable with the whole of actuality. . . I can bear to live in my own fashion, I am happy and satisfied, but my joy is not the joy of faith, and by comparison with that, it is unhappy. (34)

Abraham arouses fear and trembling in Silentio not only because Abraham challenges the efficacy of his writing-enabled reason, but because Abraham's dancing seems to realize in greater measure than Silentio's writing the joy and happiness Silentio himself seeks in making the movement of infinite resignation. In this way, the movement that makes Silentio a writer is one that binds him in bafflement to Abraham, marking both the likeness and the distance between them, enabling recognition and appreciation but not understanding.

The extent of the predicament faced by a person intending to theorize a critical affirmation of religion appears in Silentio's response to his own bafflement: he remains faithful to his "God" and writes. Yet, the more Silentio writes, the more disturbing Abraham appears. He can delineate the shape of the paradox Abraham lives, distinguish Abraham's conflicting loves, and even formulate the kind of movements that must be true for Abraham to hold onto both loves. However, whenever he tries to articulate how Abraham enters and dwells within the terms of the paradox, his rational thinking wraps itself in knots. Silentio tries at least three different approaches in

Problems I, II, and III by approaching Abraham through a concept of the ethical as the universal, a concept of God as Absolute Good, and a concept of language as a conduit of communication, respectively. How can a person welcome a call to transgress the ethical order as proof of his absolute relation to God? How can she experience the fear and trembling of doing so as a heightened enjoyment of this life? What impels an individual to invest his attention and energy in a belief that God cares about his individual well-being? From each standpoint, however, Abraham's willingness to kill Isaac for God appears absurd. Silentio can find no exit, no way to recommend this course of action to other humans. Instead of facilitating an understanding of Abraham such that he can move on, Silentio's writing produces the opposite effect: it accentuates his difference from Abraham, exacerbates his anxiety, and binds him closer to his own writing process for the admittedly small satisfaction it provides.

As he continues to write, however, Silentio knows that he is not engaging in the kind of philosophical writing Hegel describes. At various moments in the text, Silentio likens himself to a poet. When the poet looks at Abraham, he does not see spirit. Or rather, in trying to see spirit, he sees dancing—an activity that realizes the dialectical interplay of reason and experience in an opposite direction to the vector realized in philosophical writing. Where Hegel frames writing as an activity in which an *experience-enabled reason* overcomes the distinction between reason and experience, Kierkegaard frames dancing as a *reason-enabled experience*, a "later immediacy" whose meaning lies in the living and doing and having of it. Silentio and Abraham, taken separately, represent the opposing movements implied by Hegel's dialectic. Silentio's writing, even if poetic, privileges reason in its ability to overcome its difference from experience; it expresses his movement of infinite resignation. It also, however, represents a use of reason that does not lay claim to overcoming its difference from faith. Silentio cannot write across the distance he perceives between his writing reason and Abraham's dancing faith. Only Abraham is able to make both movements and somehow reconcile them within his heart. How he does so remains a mystery to Silentio and, so it seems, to anyone who writes.

Nevertheless, by writing about his bafflement, Silentio does learn; what he learns is why he cannot write Abraham's experience of faith into rational terms. The problem is not that writing is limited in relation to something like Schleiermacher's pre-reflective sensory immersion in the creative gifting of the universe. Abraham has made the movement of infinite resignation; he can think and speak about his God. Rather, Silentio learns that faith entails a reason-enabled experience that changes a person's being in the world. In that experience, reason appears in paradoxical form—as individual, singular, contextualized. Experience likewise appears as informed by and generative of concepts of space, time, community, person, human, and God. Where the practice of writing works to enforce the distinction of these two faculties (with one prevailing) in a way that ensures their reconciliation, the practice of faith as dancing cultivates the interdependence of these two faculties in a way that articulates their mutual independence.

In other words, what Silentio comes to appreciate in the effort to write about dance is how writing itself is a discipline, one that educates his desires and exercises a certain range of perceptive capacity. Silentio learns how attached he has become to the kind of thinking which writing yields in him and its pleasures. It is because he loves writing that he is amazed by Abraham—amazed that Abraham is willing to throw away the consolation and security of infinite resignation and immerse himself in the vicissitudes of worldly desire. For Silentio to make such a leap of faith would be to lose his primary source of happiness—his desire and ability to write. Why dance when you can write, reasonably, and be guaranteed its satisfactions?

In *Fear and Trembling*, then, Kierkegaard depicts "religion" as a problem that arises in the relationship between the unique, self-constituting, and irreconcilable acts of two distinct individuals: one who writes, one who dances. The poet cannot understand faith because he cannot make the leap; the dancer who makes the leap has no interest in understanding faith because faith does not appear to him as a problem. There can be no matrix or method or rational concept capable of mediating between the writer who sees faith and the dancer who does it.[10] In such a situation, to try to understand faith—or religion—would require trying to comprehend how and why and with what effects one person and not another comes to experience one thing and not another as having meaning at all. As we shall see, such is van der Leeuw's intent.

WRITING AGAINST THEOLOGY

Even though Silentio acknowledges his predicament and the impossibility of writing about faith, he cannot *not* write. In clinging to writing for the satisfaction it affords, Silentio comes to believe that writing about what cannot be written is both inevitable and necessary. Writing about faith (as he does) is *inevitable* because in an age enamored with reason, faith appears as a challenge to the scientific paradigm. Writing about faith is *necessary*, in the same breath, in order to resist "theology." In his reliance on writing to legislate an enabling resistance to theology, Silentio aligns with the philosophers and theologians he also criticizes.

Silentio's critique of theology is twofold. First, as suggested in the earlier quotation, Silentio rehearses Hegel's lament: theologians are selling religion short by trying to be like philosophers. In an attempt to offer rational defenses of religion, they mistake faith as something that has its value in moving beyond it towards enlightenment. As a result, Silentio concludes, it is necessary to write about faith in order to ensure that theologians do not cede the terms of the debate over religion to the authority of scientific culture. Like Hegel, Silentio wants to protect theology and thus religion from being explained away in rational terms.

At the same time, Silentio adds an element to Hegel's discussion that echoes Schleiermacher's critique of Kant. Silentio writes as well to unmask the theological bent of those "despisers" who presume to write as a way to secure a rational science of religion over and against "theology." Said otherwise, the theological blunder that most troubles him is not presuming some concept of the absolute or sacred (e.g., spirit for Hegel, God for Descartes, or Absolute Goodness and Truth for Kant, etc.), but presuming a transcendental method—that is, presuming that the practice of writing can ensure commensurability between rational reflection and faith. Silentio protests. Even while writing may exercise the capacity to think about spirit, the act of writing does not explain why people who can think about spirit choose to leap into the world in which spirit is their name for truth. In fact, the practice of writing and the belief in writing encourage people to forget that the question of entry is even important. So Silentio writes, for himself, to remember. In a paradigm that privileges writing as the medium of knowledge, the absence of what cannot appear in writing—the dancing—must be defended against erasure.

What initially appears as a distance between Hegel and Kierkegaard in relation to writing thus reveals a similarity as well. For each thinker, it is the act of writing—whether philosophical or poetic—that authorizes the one who writes to evaluate theology. For both, a writer is one who exercises reason over and against experience to such a degree that she makes the movement of infinite resignation. In so doing, both the philosopher and the poet participate in the life of religion—as self-consciousness of spirit or as knight of infinite resignation, respectively. In each case, it is this participation via writing in religion that gives them authority vis-à-vis theology. Hegel's philosopher is a writer who knows herself in and through writing as actualizing religion, doing the work of spirit-becoming; Silentio's poet is a writer who appreciates Abraham because he moves part way along an arc of faith he knows he cannot achieve. In both cases, writing secures the proper relationship between theory and theology—one in which theology will not collapse into philosophy, nor philosophy defer to theology. Writing negotiates their conflicted interdependence.

In sum, in his account of Silentio's frustration in writing about Abraham's dancing faith, Kierkegaard paints a picture of a predicament that haunts any project endeavoring to define and study dance as religion. Where the goal of studying religion is to translate what initially appears as non-rational (whether supernatural, theological, absurd, or incapable of empirical verification) into rational expressions (whether ethical, universal, speculative, linguistic, or logical), then the conditions that make the study of religion possible and desirable render it, at the same time, impossible. What people must do in order to prove the value of their insights as objective and rational precludes understanding religion on its own terms. Its terms become the problem to be explained or interpreted into forms that make sense to inhabitants of scientific culture. Yet, the distinctive cast of these terms as *requiring entrance*—as meaning something to someone that does not appear as "rational"—is, at the same time, what calls attention to the phenomenon as meriting explanation or interpretation. Thus, if the terms of religion can be translated, the field loses its distinctive status: it fails to demonstrate how the study of religion differs from other fields, such as anthropology, sociology, psychology, literature, history, etc., all of whom study the phenomena of religion. If they cannot be translated, the field loses its credibility as a field of scholarship. If scholars choose to believe in the fit between religion and the study of it as a way to ensure objectivity, they betray a theological entrance—a belief that whatever lies at the core of religion can be translated into conceptual form. Yet any attempt to defend the autonomy of religion vis-á-vis the study of it reflects an equally theological belief that what lies at the core of religion is something irreducible. In short, any impulse to eradicate "theology" reinscribes it, and reinforces a reliance upon the practice of writing as its primary line of defense.

As Kierkegaard's use of Silentio suggests, this whole network of issues is only compounded when the religious phenomenon in question is a dance. It is the effort to write about dance, in fact, that brings this nexus into view as a problem.

Conclusion to Part One
Living the Legacy

In the web woven from the works of these five thinkers an alternative narrative of the study of religion appears that serves to explain the popularity of the emergence narrative, the self-perpetuating antitheology polemics of the contemporary scene, the kind of attention paid to dance in the field, and their necessary interconnection.

The alternative narrative is one in which conflict with "theology" is a necessary and enabling condition for the definition and study of religion. The modern use of the term "religion" as a category of cross-cultural analysis arises coextensive with a strategy for stabilizing a contradiction between critique and affirmation embedded within the project. That strategy involves making a distinction between the study of religion and theology, and critiquing the latter. "Theology," as the story goes, speaks for a particular religious tradition and stakes its claim to truth on authorities that are not accountable to the needs and conditions of reason in its progress towards enlightenment. Attempts to theorize religion fan fears of theology when they drift too far in the direction of critique—by privileging some kind of reason over experience—or too far in the direction of affirmation—by privileging some form of experience over reason. Thus, to make a claim as to whether religion (or the quality that identifies a phenomenon as religious) is *either* reducible *or* irreducible to a process of translation into rational terms is to fall prey to "theology" as it is defined by members of the field who lean in the other direction. Furor over which vector prevails reinforces the common assumption that emergence from theology is the primary issue. Most often, at some point in their arguments, theorists on either side appeal to the practice of writing as the key to ensuring that their theories maintain the relation to theology they desire.

A narrative of conflicted interdependence or generative tension acknowledges the validity of both points of view: objective approaches to the study of religion *do* strip particular moments of phenomenal life of their particularity, and interpretive or humanistic approaches *are* biased by the participation of the subject. However, in the narrative of generative tension, the relation between theory and theology is not static. The process of contesting "theology" is not only predicted by the history of the term "religion" itself, it is a necessary condition for the vitality and growth of religious studies. The study of religion secretes suspicion of theology as a correlate of its push for academic standing. Yet those who turn against theology and rely on writing to secure an objective study for the field, fail to appreciate how the relationship between theory and theology must move in two directions. By constantly repeating the critique of theology, theorists of religion catalyze increasing self-consciousness among those doing theology about what constitutes "good" theology. Their renewed efforts, in turn, generate new material for which a writer's theories of religion must account. It is only when theology is locked in opposition to theoretical approaches that theology becomes what the writers we read resisted.

Thus a narrative of generative tension suggests that an over-reliance on writing to guarantee objectivity in religious studies serves to exacerbate rather than quell antitheology polemics that characterize the field of religious studies. Moreover, a near-exclusive use of writing as model and metaphor for meaning-making serves to divert scholars' attention from considering the effective contributions made by rhythmic bodily movement to religious life.

In exposing this matrix of issues, a narrative of generative tension suggests alternative strategies for conceiving and practicing religious studies. Where scholars perceive the moments of affirmation and critique as a rhythm to engage rather than a contradiction to resolve; where they frame theology as a generative partner rather than a nemesis; where they let go of the emergence narrative of the field as defining the terrain of battle, and resist reinscribing a faith in the practice of writing as capable of bridging the space between religion and the study of it, then they may open the possibility for attending to the action of dancing as a medium of religious experience and expression and a resource for theorizing religion.

DANCE AS RELIGION

A dancer appears. He appears to figure the impossibility of producing a science of religion capable of translating religion into concepts that make sense to those enamored with scientific culture. His appearance in this case is helpful, though troublesome. The dancer's appearance illuminates the obstacles to overcome.

For one, in the case of Silentio, the image of dancing that is produced and generated through the practice of writing is one of opposition to writing—dance appears as what writing is not. Its positive contribution to knowledge is to demonstrate the limits of writing by resisting translation into words. It does so by "fleshing out" the vector of the dialectic between reason and experience that generates experience. Yet, when the value of dance appears as the "non" to writing, attempts to take dance seriously as religion hit an impasse. To acknowledge a phenomenon that appears to defy translation into a verbal form as religion is to call into question theories and methods of studying religion founded on the belief that the dialectical relationship between reason and experience can be reconciled in writing. In so far as members of the field perceive the genesis of the study of religion as one of emerging from theology, then they will resist developing critical theories and methods capable of addressing the direction of the dialectic between reason and experience which cannot be actualized in writing—that direction illustrated by Silentio's dancing Abraham.

At the same time, the appearance of dance in Kierkegaard's text also offers hope. Kierkegaard's juxtaposition of Silentio's writing and Abraham's dancing is not a simple opposition. It reveals writing, like dancing, as itself an embodied practice. Both writing and dancing are human activities requiring rational, emotional, and sensory investment. Their difference lies in how they exercise the human faculties of reasoning and sensing in the appreciation of religion. From this perspective, a one-sided perception of their relationship as mere antithesis fails to capture Kierkegaard's insight: philosophical writing is not a question of manipulating symbolic representations. It is itself a disciplinary practice, one that educates our capacities for perception, and thus opens and forecloses avenues of understanding. Nor does dancing appear as a purely nonverbal action; it represents a later immediacy, enabled and informed by verbal practices.

In sum, Kierkegaard's juxtaposition of writing and dancing suggests that the two are in some sense mutually implicated in the study of religion. It suggests that theoretical and practical conceptions of writing and of dancing (in the modern Christian West at the very least) generate each other, and always have. His work suggests that cultivating this interdependence in some way may provide a key to realizing the potency of each medium in its distinctive contributions to theorizing religion. Perhaps we can practice writing as a form of dancing.[1] Perhaps we can thereby produce theories of language and writing more conducive to appreciating dancing as a medium of religious experience and expression and a resource for developing theory and method in the field. Part 2 sets the stage for such developments.

Part Two
REVIVING VAN DER LEEUW

G erardus van der Leeuw was a scholar with an uncanny sense of the importance of dance for religion and for the study of religion. He was also a scholar who acknowledged the impossibility of excluding "theology" from the field of religious studies. His response to the latter addressed his concern for the former. Van der Leeuw devised his phenomenology of religion as an "indirect method" for mediating the projects of historical and theological studies. In using his method, he produced some of the most original insights to date on religion and dance.

In designing his phenomenology of religion, van der Leeuw's intention was not to offer a definitive method capable of replacing or subsuming all others. Nor did he intend to offer one possibility among others in a multidisciplinary model. Van der Leeuw envisioned his phenomenology of religion as a mediating thread, weaving among "theological" approaches that stake a claim to truth and "historical" approaches of social scientific or humanist bent that detail what "is." He devised his phenomenology to help scholars regardless of approach reflect upon the assumptions informing their use of the term "religion." To this end, van der Leeuw's phenomenologist practices a dialectical movement between reason and experience and generates insights into "religion," a term whose authority resides in an ongoing process of correction by theological and historical perspectives. Van der Leeuw's willingness to choreograph a contesting, contested role for theology in religious studies provides him with a basis for critiquing theological and antitheological biases in religious studies that divert attention from dance as religion. How he orchestrates his conclusions comprises the rest of Part 2.

CHAPTER 5

A Braided Approach to the Study of Religion

Gerardus van der Leeuw

In order to appreciate the contemporary relevance of van der Leeuw's braided methodological approach to the study of religion, this chapter introduces the influences and issues informing its development. What we find is that van der Leeuw's strategies for addressing the issues of his day are relevant for our day based on the ways in which they engage and advance the issues rehearsed in Part 1 as defining the field of religious studies. Not only does van der Leeuw's work provide resources for negotiating a conflicted interdependence of theory and theology, as this chapter explores, it does so, as later chapters reveal, in ways that enable him to generate theoretical resources for understanding moments in history where dance, as rhythmic bodily movement, appears as making an effective contribution to our understanding of religion.

DEFIANT MEMORY

The life and work of Gerardus van der Leeuw defy attempts to remember him. Over the course of a relatively short life (1890-1950) van der Leeuw wrote over 650 books, articles, and review essays in three languages (Dutch, German, and French) and for three disciplines (history of religions, phenomenology of religion, and theology), addressing their respective constituencies. Only two of his major works have been translated into English.[1] He served as a pastor in the Dutch Reformed Church (1916-18), as a professor of History of Religion and the History of the Doctrine of God in the Department of Theology at the University of Groningen (1918-50), and as the Minister of Education, Arts, and Sciences in the post-World War II Dutch cabinet (1945-6).[2] As a professor, van der Leeuw taught a range of subjects, from liturgics and church history to Egyptian and Classical religions. Throughout his life, whether serving church, university, or government, he remained theologian, cultural critic, and avid musician. Although he received offers to teach elsewhere, including the Universities of Chicago and Marburg, van der Leeuw chose to stay in Groningen and actively pursue his commitment to enriching the social, cultural, religious, and intellectual lives of his own country.[3]

Attempts to consolidate the "appalling diversity of his production" are further complicated by van der Leeuw's relationship to the intellectual currents of his time.[4] Van der Leeuw came of age with the emergence narrative during the years between World Wars I and II. Scholars representing *Religionswissenschaft* were keen to emancipate the study of religion from departments of theology and secure a place for it in the academy as a science—a distinct method of knowing a particular kind of truth. Yet, as the philosophical discussions in earlier chapters predict, participants in these discussions passionately disagreed as to the terms of this transition. Some scholars advocated importing categories from the disciplines of sociology, psychology, or anthropology in order to establish an objective "science" of religion;[5] others lamented that such strategies denied "religion" any distinctive status, reducing it to a sociological, psychological, or anthropological—in effect, secular—artifact.

Within these debates, van der Leeuw was sympathetic to both perspectives and thus scorned by representatives of each. He was trained as historian of religions, studying Egyptian religions under the guidance of Chantapie de la Saussaye and Brede Kristensen, and writing a dissertation examining images of God present in texts excavated from Egyptian pyramids.[6] As he confirms, "Egyptian religion was thus my point of departure that I took care never to lose from view."[7] Upon graduating from the University of Leiden in 1916, he pastored a church, wrote *Historisch Christendom* ("Historical Christianity"), and continued his research into the religions of ancient Greece and Rome.[8] In 1918, when hired to a full professorship in a department of theology, he drew from this dual experience, moving between historical and theological approaches in giving his address: "The Place and Task of History of Religions in Theological Scholarship."[9]

It was not until 1924 that he published his so-called "little phenomenology" in Dutch, *Inleiding tot de godsdienstgeschiedenis* (Haarlem), seeking in phenomenology a way to mediate the distinction between theology and the divergent scientific studies of religion as mutually beneficial. These efforts culminated in his 1933 *Phänomenologie der Religion* (Tubingen), published in German, and translated into English in 1938 complete with an "Author's Note" giving the translation his stamp of approval.[10] As Waardenburg describes, under the banner of the "phenomenology of religion" van der Leeuw waged battle on several fronts: he fought for a "certain rehabilitation of religion against the onslaught of critical scholarship, secularization, and the rise of secular political ideologies up to 1939" on the one hand, and against theological determination on the other.[11] He sought to devise a theory and method adequate to studying whatever it was about phenomena that made them eligible for the name "religion." What he sought to know about such phenomena was something other than that guaranteed by principles of social scientific verification, or authorized by doctrine and tradition.[12] He sought understanding—understanding of the meaning that a phenomenon has for a practitioner as a function of the meaning that meaning has for the scholar. In these efforts van der Leeuw was a pioneer, rebuked by his contemporaries as both too theological and insufficiently

Christian. Nevertheless, as Eric Sharpe notes, "between 1925 and 1950, the phenomenology of religion was associated almost exclusively with the name of the Dutch scholar Gerardus van der Leeuw."[13]

Even so, van der Leeuw's contributions to the field were overshadowed by the trajectory of religious studies in Holland after his death. Interestingly enough, one of his last acts before he died was to approve the dissertation of his student, F. Sierksma, in which Sierksma attempted to "liberate" van der Leeuw's phenomenology from theological impulses. While Sierksma was hired to teach at the University of Leiden, Th. P. von Baaren was named to succeed van der Leeuw at Groningen. Still new to his position, von Baaren published an article dismissing his predecessor's phenomenology as uncritical scholarship—or (in the words of Ugo Bianchi) as "irrationalism with a protestant bias."[14] Until von Baaren's death in 1989, his view of van der Leeuw prevailed.

Together, then, Sierksma and von Baaren came to represent the kind of social science approach to *Religionswissenschaft* which van der Leeuw intended his phenomenology of religion to complement and constrain. As Waardenburg wryly notes:

> *Religionswissenschaft* was finally emancipated from theological concerns . . . by Th. P. van Baaren [in Groningen] and F. Sierksma in Leiden who, however, somewhat overdid things, as tends to happen in emancipatory processes. They naively assumed that phenomenological research as such was tainted with theology and that it could not meet scholarly standards; thus they threw out phenomenological research altogether from their concepts of an autonomous science of religions.[15]

In Waardenburg's reading, van der Leeuw was one of a cluster of exceptional individuals practicing the phenomenology of religion whose recognition and respect were largely based on their charismatic personalities and intuitive strengths.[16] Failing to establish a common method, practice, or pool of knowledge for the phenomenology of religion, van der Leeuw's "day was over, rather abruptly" at his death in 1950.[17]

The analysis from Chapters 1 through 4 suggests a complementary explanation of van der Leeuw's fall: attempts to remember van der Leeuw suffer from the polarization of the current field—already evident in his day—along antitheological lines. Van der Leeuw embraces both moments of affirmation and critique traced by the dialectic of reason and experience as integral to the task of religious studies. He does not claim to reconcile or resolve them by privileging one form of reason or experience over another in order to secure objectivity. He acknowledges this tension as a paradox embedded in the field—an irreducible tension between the claims of religion and the claims of scholarship held together in the relationship of an individual scholar to the religious phenomena that appear to her. For him, as the following sections argue, the challenge for a scholar is to sustain this paradox, and the key lies in participating in an ongoing mutual critique between theologians and historians of religions, mediated by phenomenological perspectives. It is because the chasm between history of religions and theology which van der Leeuw intentionally straddled plagues scholars of religion to this day that remembering his braided approach to the study of religion is so contested, and so valuable.[18]

SCHOLARLY CONFESSIONS

Clues to the origins of van der Leeuw's phenomenology of religion appear in his aptly, and perhaps ironically, titled *Confession Scientifique*. In this paper, van der Leeuw traces the evolution of his approach to his frustrations as a young scholar, stretched between theological claims and commitments, and his work in the history of religions (CS 8-15). Nowhere did van der Leeuw find theoretical or methodological support for making sense of the enriching effect he experienced in both his theological and historical work as a result of his movement between the two. In his estimation, attempts to define a scientific or interpretive method for grounding the study of religion over and against theology were producing an over-reliance on method as a guarantor of "objective" results. As he notes in a lecture from 1926:

> Reality should no longer be violated by forcing it, with considerable difficulty, into a purely methodological strait-jacket and then, with no less difficulty, trying to wrest it free from it after having it duly "explained" . . . reality is too rich and too manifold to leave us even the slightest hope that we may ever be able to interpret it out of one single principle and by one single method.[19]

When a scholar allows a conceptual scheme to dominate his interaction with the material of religious life, he narrows and slants his vision of the rich manifold of the given such that his findings say more about the method used than about the manifold under consideration. For this reason, van der Leeuw rejected the "imperiously dominating" theories of his day associated with Primal Dynamism, Animism, or Monotheism (REM xxi); he criticized attempts to explain religion as an entity whose unity is given by some *historical* origin, primal cause, or developmental track, especially when that explanation was recycled to ground an evaluation of particular religious truths with respect to one another. It is scholars taking such historical and theological approaches, he affirmed, who bind "reality" into a "methodological straight jacket," forcing the facts to fit the theory and losing the particular objects under consideration.

This critique, in itself, is familiar to us from the analysis in Part 1. All of the thinkers discussed were concerned at one time or another with affirming the particularity of religious phenomena in the face of philosophical argument. Van der Leeuw's response, by contrast, is not to offer a better theory of religion per se, but rather to develop guidelines for helping religionists—whether historians or theologians—to take adequate account of whatever presuppositions enable and delimit their conception of "religion." In this regard, van der Leeuw was reluctant even to call his phenomenology of religion a "method"; he preferred, for reasons that will emerge, the term "indirect method" (REM 677-8).

In designing his indirect method, van der Leeuw sought an "orientation" or "perspective" that would enable him to think critically about why one phenomenon and not another appears as religion; in other words, how such a phenomenon shows itself to us [*comme il se montre à nous*] as religion. As his *Confession* explains:

> I always greatly felt a need to find a means for embracing all of the vast domain of world religions, without being restricted to several areas whose language and civilization were accessible to me, and without, meanwhile, losing myself in a poorly grounded dilettantism. And behind this need for orientation and perspective, I felt more and more a need to penetrate to the heart of this impressive and enigmatic phenomenon, religion, to find the path which leads from the scattered, semi-detached phenomena of historical religions to the essence of the phenomenon, to proceed from religions to religion, to its being as it reveals itself to us.[20]

For van der Leeuw, religion is not an actual entity existing in time and space. Religion is a *phenomenon*— "that which appears"—arising in the relationship between individuals and what they perceive. The "religion" van der Leeuw seeks is not a concrete, historical body of evidence nor a perennial philosophy; it does not refer to either the sum of all religions, nor one great unifying spring from which all other religions emanate. Religion refers to a term, an imaginative schema that enables the perception and study of myriad phenomena. It is a conceptual sieve that allows scholars to distinguish one thing and not another as capable of being explained in relation to other things appearing to share similar distinguishing qualities. As such, van der Leeuw seeks a method that will help scholars grasp the meaning of the term "religion" as a "path" that weaves in and through their own theological evaluations and historical studies of diverse and disparate moments of human existence. By directing reflection on the meaning of this term, van der Leeuw intends to serve theologians and historians of various shades in improving their respective projects.

This goal qualifies what van der Leeuw means when he claims to seek the "essence" of "religion": that essence is an appearance. It is a function of the relationship between the person to whom an appearance happens and the qualities of that which appears. From the outset, van der Leeuw denies that scholars have access to some Other reality behind the forms which appear to them as religion; he denies that there is one definition of religion which can or will fulfill this conceptual function for all people or all religion as phenomena. Instead he acknowledges an indissoluble unity of a researcher's experience and the artifact observed— "de la vie et du vécu" or "of life and the lived"—as the relational context within which religion appears.[21] It is in this sense that van der Leeuw describes "religion" as a "path [*chemin*]." It represents the conceptual journey scholars make as they pass among scattered historical reference points, connecting them through their imaginative movement as sharing a kind of meaning.

Searching for resources adequate to investigating the conditions between scholar and culture which catalyze appearances of religion, van der Leeuw looked to the history of religions, structural psychology, the social sciences, theology, art, music, and literature before leaving them behind and setting out to develop what he called a "phenomenology of religion" (CS 10).

DISCIPLINARY INTERPLAY

In van der Leeuw's hands, the phenomenology of religion arises as a mediating thread between the disciplines of theology, on the one hand, and the social scientific and humanist approaches to the study of religion (a group I am loosely calling "historians"), on the other.

Van der Leeuw's insistence that the strands of this disciplinary braid cannot be unraveled, dissolved, or systematized into a single method is unique. For him, no one of the disciplines can stand alone as an authority. Together, they represent a play of tensions, a system of checks and balances whose extension delineates the width, length, and depth of the field of religious studies. A brief look at how the disciplines enable and constrain one another provides the context for a closer look at the mediating work of his phenomenological method in Chapter 6.

In this braid, the interdependence of two of the strands—historical projects and the phenomenology of religion—is easiest to grasp. As van der Leeuw describes, any move to name a historical moment of religion and frame one's analysis of it as relevant for understanding religion—regardless of the social science or interpretive stance invoked—presupposes some concept of "religion" in general such that the moment can appear as one example. Such a category, on the one hand, enables a historian to affirm the sensorial particularity of the moment as religion, yet, on the other, does so effectively only by relying on some standard grounded on a basis apart from the givens of the historical case. The use of that standard may be justified in different ways, as we have seen in Part 1—for example, by appeal to rational methods, or to a believer's experience, or to a concept of spirit. Regardless, as van der Leeuw confirms, the most purely empirical attention to facts as relevant to the study of *religion* depends upon a notion of religion not given by those particulars. Any description of what happened is not possible "without the naming, without the choice, without the penetration with the help of introspection that comprises, in their combination, the phenomenological method."[22]

Correlatively, where phenomenological concepts such as "religion" enable historical inquiry, the use of those concepts qualifies the kinds of claims historians or cultural interpreters can make about what they notice. A "fact" about religion is never and can never be purely objective given that it is mediated by an *understanding* of what religion is. To

the extent that an historical description of religion presumes phenomenological concepts, van der Leeuw attests, any "fact" about religion is never a concretely present "reality."[23]

Where historical study is enabled and constrained by phenomenology, the reverse is true as well. Van der Leeuw acknowledges
that a phenomenologist cannot begin to formulate an understanding
of religion capable of orienting historical study without moving
across the terrain of historical examples provided by historians. He
writes:

> The phenomenologist is bound up with the object; he cannot
> proceed without repeatedly confronting the chaos of the given,
> and without submitting again and again to correction by the
> facts . . . his path lies always between the unformed chaos of the
> historical world and its structural endowment with form. All his
> life he oscillates hither and thither. (REM 685-6)

While the historian, hedged by empirical methods, stands still before
an historical event, resigning herself to "establishing what has actually happened," even if it means mere cataloguing and description
(REM 686), the phenomenologist moves constantly across the
"unformed chaos" of history, ever willing to submit to historical
objects even as he endlessly turns away from the particular cases,
seeking to recreate the forms of their appearance. So intertwined are
the tasks of history and phenomenology, van der Leeuw argues, that
"they are indeed in the majority of cases combined in the person of a
single investigator" (REM 686).

Yet, despite the swirling intimacy of these projects, van der Leeuw
maintains their difference: while an historian of religions aims to
establish, explain, and/or interpret what happened, a phenomenologist of religion seeks to understand how and why what happened registers as "religion." Historical approaches to religions presuppose a
degree of phenomenological understanding, and phenomenology
requires constant correction by historical examples; yet, the two

remain distinct concerning the questions posed and goals pursued in relation to the "unformed chaos" of human worlds.

The theological strand within van der Leeuw's braided approach to the study of religions is as entwined with the phenomenology of religion and the history of religions as these two are with one another. Alone among those engaged in religious studies, van der Leeuw confirms, a theologian speaks from and for a particular religious tradition, intentionally hazarding judgments as to the truth and value of its forms and contents in relation to those of other traditions. Even so, he explains, the ability to make such proclamations depends upon sound historical accounts and phenomenological understandings of what a particular doctrine or belief or practice is and means, has been and has meant, in history. Comprehending the degree of interdependence van der Leeuw observes between theology and other disciplines requires spending a few paragraphs elucidating van der Leeuw's conception of what it means to speak from and for a tradition as a theologian.[24]

UNMASKING THEOLOGY

Van der Leeuw's own definition of theology represents what he has learned from nineteenth-century critics of theology, including those described in Part 1. His definition incorporates their critiques in a way that both distinguishes theology from the history and phenomenology of religion and acknowledges its importance as a generative partner in religious studies. It is contestation with theology, van der Leeuw insists, that marks these other non-theological approaches to the study of religion as studying *religion*.

Theology, van der Leeuw admits, speaking under the influence of Christian theology, begins with faith—the faith that God communicates with human beings through forms accessible to human experience. Van der Leeuw does not address the (Hegel/ Kierkegaard) question of whether faith is an originary or later immediacy. He affirms that either way, faith appears in relation to historical forms of religion—that, for a person with faith, mediate a relation to that in which a person has faith—for example, "God." At the same time, he continues, the work of theology presupposes reason as well; it consists in "reflecting" upon these historical forms and seeking to comprehend what God is or is not communicating through them. In their reflections, theologians aspire to science: they proceed rationally, through observation, classification, and the application of logical principles. Succinctly stated: "Theology is science which preaches, Preaching which reflects. It preaches that God has directed Himself towards this world. It reflects on the forms which this act of God has assumed in the life of the world."[25] By defining theology as engaging both the experience of faith and the practices of science, van der Leeuw identifies theology as participating in the same dialectical tension between experience and reason we have observed as driving the study of religion in general.

Van der Leeuw elaborates this conception of theology by reflecting upon what he as a Christian theologian identifies as the paradigmatic act of communication—the communication between human and "God" figured by the Christian Incarnation. He explains:

> Truth is only in communication. . . . The theological name for communication is Incarnation. And the Incarnation is the presupposition for every communication among men. Here—and here alone—is the Dogma of the Church. . . . Dogma is . . . the living reality of communication between Christ and his Church which is given with the Incarnation. Thus, there is really only one dogma: God became man; all other doctrines are valid only in so far as the Theologia dogmatica can derive them from the one.[26]

Here, van der Leeuw seems to fall prey to the critique of his philosophical forebears who accuse theologians of appealing to an authority beyond reason and then elevating that authority above all others as the standard of accountability—the "one dogma." From their perspective, a theologian who makes such an appeal disqualifies himself from any role in a scientific study of religion; any insights he produces will not be accountable to the needs of reason reflecting upon experience.

At the same time that he insists that theology begins with faith, van der Leeuw nevertheless challenges the idea that theology is *fixed* by this faith in a communicative God. On the contrary: theology, he concedes, is effective only in so far as a theologian acknowledges with every turn of phrase that communication between God and human is never assured and never complete. The forms of God's communication are not God; analysis of these forms can never deliver God; if they could deliver God, there would be no God communicating through them. In van der Leeuw's words:

> A Dogmatics which attempts this task [of deriving all doctrines from the Incarnation] must share in the communication, that is to say, it must be an act of faith . . . This act is never completed. Again and again it fails. Were it to succeed, then there would have disappeared from Theology the tension in which we recognize the basic structure of Incarnation, then it would no longer be Incarnation theology. But incomplete, strong in faith, it moves in the Church, apostolic and catholic, as the act of all the members.[27]

By insisting that the faith with which theology begins is a faith in *communication* rather than in a particular Being per se, van der Leeuw sidesteps the critiques of theology discussed in Part 1. For him, theology participates in an irreducible tension: it is suspended between a need to articulate the difference between human and God that makes communication possible, desirable, and worth interpreting, on the one hand, and the promise of communion between human and God on the other. The faith with which theology begins predicts that an analysis of worldly forms will yield an understanding of God, and that God is necessarily absent from those forms. Both contradictory statements must be true in order for God to be God for humans. The implication for a theologian is this: only by acknowledging her failure to deliver knowledge of God can a theologian allow for the possibility that those forms may actually be of God—that God is—that God is something Other towards which the forms gesture. In so far as a theologian acknowledges that her work is "never completed" and that her words can never make God present, then her theological writing succeeds in manifesting the "structure of Incarnation": she makes visible a double movement in which God appears moving towards humans while humans move towards God, meeting in the forms of God's communicating Word. Van der Leeuw's theologian begins to resemble Kierkegaard's dancer.

For van der Leeuw, this tension between the necessity and the impossibility of theology manifests as an "eternal dynamic," binding as members of a community all those who engage in ongoing efforts to name and enact the forms of God's incarnating activity. Theology thus entails the "scientific discovery of the movement [*dynamis*] of the dogma of the Church."[28]

THEOLOGY ENTWINED

With this definition of theology as a dynamic, incomplete, ongoing reflection on the forms of "God"'s appearing, van der Leeuw unmasks the specter that haunts attempts to theorize religion. Theologians, he claims, participate in the same dialectical rhythm between reason and experience as do scholars of religion. As such, not only do theologians need the historical (social science and humanist) and phenomenological perspectives in order to do better theology, these approaches in turn need theology to evaluate and critique the truth claims smuggled in to their respective stances.

First, theology as van der Leeuw envisions it does not threaten to arrest the free play of reason or occlude ongoing receptivity to experiences of infinity; rather, it involves applying reason to interpret what a theologian believes are forms of God's incarnating activity. That any given form is presumed to communicate God marks a judgment specific to the theologian, predicated on faith. However, that judgment also presupposes an informed recognition of possible forms in and through which God might appear. Thus, a theologian draws resources from phenomenological and historical studies in order to enhance the "scientific" dimension of his work, as he describes and classifies the forms of God's communicating activity. Describing his experience, van der Leeuw writes:

> I have never felt the need to forget that I am a theologian, and naturally, I have sought to make theology profit from the phenomenological method. Not, certainly, for the purpose of making theology into a science of religion, but on the contrary, for better distinguishing the theological method which, in my opinion, is absolutely autonomous . . . In other words, phenomenology ought to help theology organize its facts, penetrate their meanings, and find in them their essences, before theology evaluates them and employs them for dogmatic purposes.[29]

Van der Leeuw is clear. Theology is not a "science of religion"; it presupposes and expresses faith. Nevertheless, a theologian fails in his attempt to "preach" if he cannot communicate with and learn from those who do not share his faith.

In addition, van der Leeuw discloses how within any attempt to draw the contours of *a* religion or claim the truth of a tradition there lurks an understanding whose basis of authority extends beyond the parameters of the one tradition to reference other religions of the world. A theologian's proclamation of the Christian message as one of incarnation, for example, is mediated by phenomenological understandings of "incarnation," "communication," "form," and "reflection," and historical examples documenting the usefulness of such categories. Even to proclaim incarnation as the "one dogma" of Christian religion requires drawing upon a matrix of phenomena to distinguish and authorize this particular phenomenon and not another as the center and source of Christian faith. In this way, van der Leeuw acknowledges with Hegel that faith is a "wholly relative moment of origin," enabled and informed by facts and concepts, the objects of historical and phenomenological studies. The forms upon which theology reflects are the forms whose existence the historian purports to verify, and the forms whose meaning as religion the phenomenologist seeks to understand. As such, these disciplines play a crucial role in both enabling and checking theological claims. In van der Leeuw's words, the role of the phenomenology of religion in relation to theology compares with the function of a South African thorn bush—the *Watchebietjie*—whose name means "wait a bit."[30]

Conversely, as theological reflection depends upon and is accountable to the phenomenological and historical study of religions, so too are these disciplines both enabled and constrained by theology. In one respect, the enabling/constraining role is evident: in studying the material, behavioral and doctrinal forms on which theologians also reflect, historians and phenomenologists are accountable to theological interpretations as signposts for religion. The fact that theological claims are made in relation to certain objects, events, and artifacts is part of what phenomenologists take into account when shaping their sense of what counts as religion, and part of what social scientists and those employing humanist approaches acknowledge in their attempt to establish the facts of religion. For van der Leeuw, what the historian can describe as a fact of religion and the phenomenologist claim as the meaning of religion appear respectively as fact and meaning in so far as the phenomenon is marked by someone—whether practitioner or scholar—as a form of Communication. Even when a social scientist intends to explain theology away as ideological illusion, she presumes that there is something that warrants explaining; her method affirms not a given faith, but the possibility that someone might have faith. In this way, the contest with theology is what differentiates social scientific, humanist, and phenomenological studies of religion as being "of religion." Their distinctive status within the university thus depends upon and is constrained by rational reflection that presupposes the existence, if not the desirability, of faith.

Further, as van der Leeuw's rendering suggests, theologians have a role to play in addressing and defusing the antitheology debates between those humanists and social scientists who promote the emergence narrative as a paradigm for the field. In so far as the task of theology is to identify the forms of God's communication as *incomplete*, theology represents a perspective able to unmask as false the theological assumptions and assumptions *about theology* embedded in the poles of the antitheological debates. In particular, van der Leeuw allies with thinkers from Part 1 suggesting that the opposition between theology and objective study is a false one: it conceals the interdependence of the two when the object in question is *religion*. Fidelity to the emergence narrative prevents scholars from appreciating and accessing their dependence on theology as an enabling and constraining influence.

Even so, van der Leeuw admits that engaging theology as a generative partner in religious studies is not without its dangers. Here the phenomenologist of religion plays a vital mediating role. By moving between theology and antitheology positions, a phenomenologist helps provide historical context for theological meanings and helps disclose the theological assumptions enabling and informing historical findings. In this winding dance, a phenomenologist helps each discipline do its work better by becoming conscious of its interdependence with the others. A phenomenologist's goal is understanding— understanding how and why and to what ends something (whether art, icon, ritual, text) appears to someone (whether inside or outside a given tradition) as relevant to understanding what the term "religion" says about it. His reflections on the concept of religion thus connect and space the projects of historical study and theological evaluation.[31]

The strands of this braided approach to the study of religions may be gathered as follows: while a description of historical moments is focused and narrowed by an understanding about what counts as "religion," and while historical accounting and phenomenological understanding both materialize and contextualize theological preaching, the need for accountability to both historical "facts" and theological "truths" checks the phenomenological understandings of religious phenomena which inform in turn historical and theological projects. A historian stands still observing; a phenomenologist moves between the "chaos of the given" and structural form, wedded to this earth; a theologian moves between the known and the unknown. Each discipline emerges as distinctive in its respective winding of the empirical, conceptual, and imaginative tasks they share and in the species of conclusions each draws about the religious lives of human beings—conclusions about fact (for history, whether explained or interpreted), meaning (for phenomenology), or truth (for theology). The movement of the phenomenologist "on earth" weaves a connective tissue among the disciplines that is stretched and strengthened in the exercise of any one of the three. As van der Leeuw claims, "Of heaven and hell, however, phenomenology knows nothing at all; it is at home on earth, although it is at the same time sustained by love of the beyond" (REM 688).

CONCLUDING NOTES

In van der Leeuw's teaching and publishing record, the interplay among these disciplines is evident. For instance, the publication of the culminating edition of his *Phänomenologie* in French in 1948 coincided with the publication of his greatest theological work, *Sacramentstheologie*, in Dutch. In this latter work, he begins his theological rendering of the Christian sacraments with a phenomenological and historical survey of "sacrament" and its various meanings, and then, in the second half, draws upon these analyses to enrich and nuance his theological reflections on the Christian case. As the analyses in Chapters 8 and 9 illustrate as well, van der Leeuw's reflections on dance as religion demonstrate his commitment to being a theologian, an historian of religions, and a phenomenologist of religion at once, and to embracing the tensions among these tasks as generative of each.

When van der Leeuw's phenomenology is accorded its mediating role in van der Leeuw's braided approach to the study of religions, it is no wonder that his work is "too easily" forgotten: his braided approach poses a radical challenge to the emergence narrative. What van der Leeuw confronts head-on and accepts is the idea that the conceptual movements required to comprehend the complexity of any one moment of religious life necessarily conflict. No single method for the study of religions, whether it sports a sophisticated method or a concern with the particularity of religious phenomena, can grasp the multiple dimensions mobilized in every application of the term "religion." Nor can a single set of criteria be drawn to which all projects in the study of religion can apply. The differences among criteria cannot be homogenized from the perspective of one of them. It is irrelevant, for example, to judge phenomenological or theological claims based on standards applicable to empirical study of "facts"— neither phenomenology or theology (as defined by van der Leeuw) intends to deliver "facts." Likewise, it is impossible to judge the accuracy of facts based on an appeal to theological truths or a definition of religion. These disciplinary angles are stubbornly heterogeneous. Even though their respective tasks, their goals and criteria implicate one another, they cannot "be brought together systematically in a unified whole."[32] They cross one another, enabling and arresting each other, with each discipline surfacing in the field of tensions they comprise as both necessary and impossible.

Here van der Leeuw has a response for his critics: those who remember him simply as a phenomenologist and dismiss his phenomenology as too theological from the point of view of empirical science profess their ignorance of what van der Leeuw creates his phenomenology of religion to be—a guide to conscious reflection upon the presumptions, limitations, and interdependence of projects in religious studies which present themselves as historical, scientific, interpretive, or theological. Such critics unravel his methodological braid and in the process, deny phenomenology its mediating role between the history of religions and theology. Scholars who miss these features are unable to set his theological claims in their relevant contexts and fail to appreciate the contributions his approach makes to debates concerning the tasks and scope of religious studies.

In offering a braided approach to the study of religion, one in which theology appears as a strand, van der Leeuw provides a way both to understand and defuse the current suspicion of theology that pits social scientific and humanistic perspectives against one another and both against theology. As we will see, he does so by encouraging scholars to practice both movements of affirmation and critique in relation to whatever appears to them as religion in order to generate understanding of it. How a scholar can do so responsibly, as Chapter 6 investigates, is the concern van der Leeuw designs his phenomenology of religion to address.

CHAPTER 6

A Practice of Understanding

In what, then, does the phenomenology of religion consist? What does it mean to call religion a *phenomenon*? Where does the phenomenologist of religion look to find "it"? What kinds of movements propel the phenomenologist back and forth across the surface of historical events, between the chaos of the given and conceptual forms? By what means does a phenomenologist mediate between the historical, scientific, and interpretive approaches to the study of religion, on the one hand, and theology on the other?

As suggested in Chapter 5, it was van der Leeuw's frustration with the chasm he perceived between historical and theological approaches to the study of religion that impelled him to distinguish a study of *religion* from the description of historical *fact* or attempts to posit *truth* as a mediating activity between the two, and correlatively, to formulate a phenomenology of religion as a means for engaging critically in that mediating activity. It is fair to say that van der Leeuw's phenomenological method and his concept of religion as a phenomenon pulled each other into existence—the one serving to articulate the other. In his own words, a phenomenon is "what appears" and phenomenology begins when a person discusses what appears (REM 671). Following his guide, this chapter enters his phenomenology through a discussion of the phenomenon.

In his conception of a phenomenon, as discussed below, the hinge of his argument for a braided methodological approach, van der Leeuw offers his response to the problematic framed by his philosophical forebears, namely, how to develop a scientific study of religion that both affirms the particularity of phenomena that appear as "religion" and allows for a critical understanding of those phenomena. He does so by defining a phenomenon as an *appearance of meaning* where that meaning appears to someone in an open-ended, mutually generative dialectic of reason and experience. His phenomenological method, in turn, takes shape as a *practice of understanding* in which scholars cultivate the ability to move between rational reflections and the appearances of meaning they experience. They do so in ways that enhance their ability to recognize and interpret such appearances as "religion." Thus, van der Leeuw seeks to articulate an approach to studying religion that nourishes the historical study of facts and the theological quest for truth without forcing an opposition between the two nor collapsing one into the other.

Along the way, the significance of van der Leeuw's phenomenology of religion for attempts to appreciate dance as a medium of religious experience and expression begins to appear: by defining and mobilizing (the relation between) reason and experience as he does, van der Leeuw's phenomenology of religion opens the possibility for approaches to studying religion that do not demand an oppositional stand in relation to "theology" and do not, correlatively, rely exclusively on writing as a model of and for knowledge. As later chapters suggest, van der Leeuw's model of and for knowing is a dialectical interplay of writing and dancing.

THE SHAPE OF A PHENOMENON

While the phrase "what appears" might seem to reference a concrete object apart from a subject, van der Leeuw maintains that "appearance" refers equally to what appears and to the person to whom it appears; the phenomenon, therefore, is neither pure object, nor *the* object, that is to say, the actual reality, whose essential being is merely concealed by the "appearing" of the appearance; with this a specific metaphysics deals. The term "phenomenon," further, does not imply something purely subjective, not a "life" of the subject; so far as is at all possible, a definite branch of psychology is concerned with this. The "phenomenon" as such, therefore, is an object related to a subject, and a subject related to an object ... [with no modification implied] ... The phenomenon ... is not produced by the subject, and still less substantiated or demonstrated by it; its entire essence is given in its "appearance," and its appearance to "someone." (REM 671)

A phenomenon is a relation: it *is* "an object related to a subject, and a subject related to an object"—something-appearing-to-someone. Both parties are necessary for the appearance to occur, both are pulled into shape by the encounter, and neither exclusively determines the content of the appearing. The phenomenon or form that appears conceals the "actual reality" of what is given because what appears appears to a particular person, as conditioned by her perceptive capabilities. On the other hand, what appears is not a subjective fiction; some *thing* appears as having a meaning apart from and in relation to a sense of self. The subject appears as subject (capable of perceiving this phenomenon) in the moment that the object appears as an object (capable of being perceived). As such, the *essence* of a phenomenon, van der Leeuw explains, is a *relation*: it is the relation that enables, constitutes, and comes into existence at the moment of an appearing. Because an essence is an appearance, it cannot be categorized as either "fact" or "truth." What appears is what an "I" can see; an "I" emerges as the one who sees what appears.

Neither subject nor object nor fusion of the two, the "essence" of a phenomenon is a "third thing," that which van der Leeuw describes as "meaning." *Meaning*, for van der Leeuw, is what "dawns upon me" in the moment something appears (REM 673). Meaning is at once *my* meaning and *its* meaning, "irrevocably one in the act of comprehension" (REM 673). In his interaction with the chaotic maze of the given, an observer experiences himself as being struck by something because some thing appears to him to *have* meaning in itself or for someone else ("its meaning"). At the same time, its meaning arises as a function of the observer's perceiving its meaning as having meaning for him—a different meaning, but meaning nonetheless ("my meaning"). In discussing what appears, then, a phenomenologist seeks to understand whatever it is about his relation to the object that enables him to experience it as having meaning for him.

Van der Leeuw develops several terms which help him map the multidimensional form of a phenomenon: structure or structural relation; ideal type; and name. All three terms describe a different set of elements necessary for a phenomenon, that is, a "third thing" or "meaning," to appear. Although, in his "Epilegomena" to *Religion in Essence and Manifestation*, van der Leeuw introduces names first, then structural relations and ideal types, he insists that, "in practice, they arise never successively but always simultaneously, and in their mutual relations far more frequently than in series" (REM 674). I will here take the liberty of beginning by discussing structures, before proceeding to discuss ideal types and names.

Structure or Structural Relation

At its most general level, a phenomenon is a *structure* or a *structural relation*. These terms are synonymous for van der Leeuw. He explains structure as follows:

> Structure is a connection which is neither merely experienced directly, nor abstracted logically or causally, but which is *understood*. It is an organic whole which cannot be analyzed into its

own constituents, but which can from these be comprehended; or in other terms, a fabric of particulars, not to be compounded by the addition of these, nor the deduction of one . . . but again only *understood* as a whole . . . Structure is reality significantly organized. (REM 672)

According to van der Leeuw, as noted above, "what appears" to be an object is not a "thing" at all; it is a nexus of relationships among many particulars, an "organic whole" comprised of "manifold individual images" (SRA 404). The particulars that comprise this fabric represent moments of the subject's experience—what she has learned and lived. Yet these experiences are not individual scraps, pieced together to make the fabric. In the moment any phenomenon appears, the fabric appears in whole cloth as the web of relationships within which that single image appears as having meaning. Part and whole appear in the same instant as a function of each other.

By defining a structure as a fabric of particulars, van der Leeuw is not suggesting that a person experiences an object because it resembles other objects—as if an object existed out there as an object ready to be compared and contrasted with other objects. His point is that something appears to someone as having a distinguishing shape, or a sensory form that serves as the quality or characteristic relating that moment to others in his history. It is such shared, familiar qualities that enable a person to notice it at all as meaning anything. In the moment of appearing, a person experiences a structural relation—the fabric of particulars that enables the appearance—and not the actual reality of some thing. Van der Leeuw's description of a phenomenon as a structural relation implies, as for Hegel and followers, that there are no pure objects nor any unmediated experiences.

Further, because a phenomenon is a structural relation, its appearance is inseparable from the self of the person to whom it appears. A person cannot coerce meaning into appearing. She can receive it, allowing structures to appear to her in relation to a given swath of human expressions by way of both her past experiences and her reflections on them. She is the fabric of particular experiences that pulls and is pulled into shape by the appearance of another person's experience to her. As van der Leeuw phrases it, any single experience of meaning "extends over several experiential unities simultaneously, as indeed it also originates from the comprehension of these unities of experience" (REM 673). Again, a person does not piece together her past experiences in response to the appearance of an "object." Rather, she can perceive something and not nothing only through its relationship with other moments of her experience. Thus, in a phenomenon, a person sees her perceptive reasoning capacity—her *self*—as extending through space and time, and constituted by a web of "experiential unities." Her sense of self is mediated by the (absence of the) object she creates herself to understand. In discussing what appears, a person casts a net over reality in which she herself is caught.

Ideal Type

When a phenomenologist perceives the structural relations girding the appearance of an object to him, and represents those structural relations in terms of a kind of object they make apparent, he articulates the "essence" of the phenomenon, in terms of what van der Leeuw calls an ideal type (*Idealtypen*) (SRA 404). Borrowing loosely from Max Weber, van der Leeuw defines ideal types as "images of the mind, which combine certain processes and relations into a unified whole" (SRA 404). Van der Leeuw's use of this term can be confusing because he does not intend to refer to an entity other than that named by "structural relation" but rather, to illuminate a different facet of a phenomenon's appearing. The terms overlap. Where van der Leeuw uses "structure" to trace the basic form of the phenomenon as a fabric of particulars, he uses the term "ideal type" to illuminate how that fabric functions in relation to the particular image that catalyzed the moment of meaning appearing. It functions as a category.

For van der Leeuw the phenomenon that appears in a given moment—because it is a structural relation—can be represented as a "type," that is, as one example of a general species. A phenomenologist can depict the fabric of particulars that appears as a given phenomenon in terms of some shared family of elements that enable the connections to form among moments of his experience. Any particular that appears as a moment in the fabric thus also appears as a representative of this type (REM 673). In this sense, "type" is another way of representing van der Leeuw's insight that every experience is always already a connection (REM 673). The identity of any "object" is at once constituted and concealed in an act of comprehension by its relationship with other objects familiar to the scholar. It acquires meaning in relation to similar objects only by losing something of its "actual reality" as a particular.

In this respect, any appearance of a given structure not only defines a *type* or category of items, it is also *ideal* in two senses. First, with this adjective "ideal," van der Leeuw emphasizes his conviction that every appearance requires investment on the part of the one to whom the appearance occurs. A type is "constructed" by the observer in order to represent her relation to the object, mediated as it is by a set of processes and past experiences. Van der Leeuw summarizes the relationship between ideal type and structure in this way:

> The ideal-typical construction may rather be compared to the products of the artistic mind, which likewise express a kind of dual experience . . . The ideal type is . . . formed indeed on the basis of experience, but it is not derived from experience—just as the hero of a drama. It must have gone through the stages of phenomenological clarification and of the formation of structural relations. Both the hero and the ideal type have as their purpose to make life intelligible by an experienced construc-

tion of normative character. The expression "experienced construction" (*erlebte Konstruktion*) as such is, of course, non-
sense. What is meant is that in experience the construction—or
rather, the *structure*—of a person, of an event, etc. becomes
"evident," "obvious." We do not "construct," but we experience a unity of meaning. It is therefore, clear that these ideal
types have no reality as little as have the essences or the structural relations . . . What matters is only their potentiality.
(SRA 405-6)

As constructions, types are "ideal" in a second way as well because
they impose an order on reality—an order that appears as a person
reflects on a phenomenon that appears to her. Types have a normative
character. Once forged as a description of a phenomenon, an ideal
type may shepherd the appearance of other phenomena, serving to
classify and organize the manifold flux of life. In this regard, van der
Leeuw stands firm: ideal types express a "dual experience." They do
not represent "life" itself, or even a "primal experience" of life, but
rather, a human reflecting on her experience of meaning in an effort
to render life intelligible. Ideal types represent a phenomenologist's
reconstruction of the structural relations that allow a phenomenon to
appear as one among many. The actual and the ideal, like the part and
(a sense of) the whole, appear at once, as a function of one another.

Here, van der Leeuw's definition of an ideal type highlights a
rhythm of action and reception in which an inquiring subject is
engaged. On the one hand, a person "constructs" these types: he
applies his reason to representing the elements shared by particulars
comprising those structural relations by means of which a phenomenon appears. On the other, the meaning he "constructs" is given
to him in his experience—that is, in the unity of its and my meaning
that occurs as a phenomenon bursts into view. Citing a Dutch theologian, van der Leeuw writes, "one takes into oneself and gives rebirth,
out of one's own mind, to what stands already there" (SRA 402). In

this process, a person formulates ideal types not to mirror the "already there" but rather to help him understand why something appears to him as "already there." As van der Leeuw concludes, what matters about an ideal type is its "potentiality." What is reborn out of one's mind must have a life of its own, giving shape to future experiences of meaning in accord with the nexus of relations it represents.

Name

When a phenomenon appears, in the form of a structural relation, defined by an ideal type, as a recreation of an appearance of meaning, a phenomenologist names it—in "fear and trembling." Van der Leeuw confides: "In the assignment of names we expose ourselves to the peril of becoming intoxicated, or at least, satisfied, with the name—the danger which Goethe represented as 'transforming observations into mere concepts, and concepts into word,' and then treating these words 'as if they were objects'" (REM 674). A name is a word attached to an image of a particular. A name can "intoxicate" because it appears as a simple, immediate reference for an evidently present object. The ease with which people name and manipulate names lulls them into forgetting that the name is not the object, and that the ability to assign a name presupposes an appearance of meaning to someone mediated by multiple layers of reflection and experience, structural relations, and ideal types. In short, names seduce people into forgetting their role and responsibility in courting appearances of meaning.

Nevertheless, van der Leeuw concedes, such naming is the goal of a phenomenologist, in particular, and of science in general. It is in and through the bestowal of names that "chaotic and obstinate 'reality' thus becomes a manifestation, a revelation . . . [T]he intangible experience in itself cannot be apprehended nor mastered, but that it manifests something to us, an appearance . . . an utterance. The aim of science, therefore, is to understand this *logos*; essentially science is hermeneutics" (REM 676). Any appearance is a manifestation; it appears as a meaning, an utterance or *logos* whose shape van der Leeuw's science seeks to read and interpret. Yet what is revealed in and through a *phenomenon* for a phenomenologist is not reality nor "intangible experience," but the conditions enabling something to appear to someone as meaning and not chaos. The "essence" a phenomenologist seeks *is* comprised of structural relations, that is, the fabrics of particulars webbing subject and object that enable a phenomenon to appear at all. Thus to name a particular is to see it as having meaning, as being intelligible, by virtue of its relations with other particulars whose appearances are woven into the structural relation the name represents. *To name is to understand.*

In her concern with phenomena, then, a phenomenologist is not interested in cataloguing the features of an utterance (as are historical approaches), or in ascertaining their claims to truth (as are theological approaches); she seeks instead to recreate for herself what that utterance means to whomever claims it as fact or truth. She asks, what does the fact of this appearing reveal? She seeks to name it, in terms of an ideal type of human phenomena. With reference to Kierkegaard, van der Leeuw asserts that a phenomenon as he defines it provides the only "entrance gate" to understanding the life of another that he can find (REM 673).

RELIGION: A PHENOMENON

Given this rendering of a phenomenon, what does it mean to identify *religion* as a phenomenon? What is the significance of such an identification?

As a phenomenon, religion is a *name* for an *ideal type* representing the *structural relations*—the fabric of particulars stretching across multiple moments of experience—that come into being for someone in the moment when he experiences something as having meaning for him by virtue of its relation to experiences he has already understood as "religion." Religion does not refer to a thing or a universal essence or a reality out there. It is a "net" or "network" which a scholar casts *over* the "chaotic maze of so-called reality" (REM 672). As a net of experiential unities tossed over the given, religion is constantly open to challenge by the particular phenomena whose appearance it makes possible. Every new toss of the term changes the composition of the web. A new particular appears in it and a scholar refines his concept of what "religion" is. His new ideal allows other phenomena to appear to him as intelligible by virtue of their relation to what is familiar to him. Thus, where religion is a phenomenon, any definition of religion is partial, provisional, and rooted in a particular relational context as is the process of understanding whatever appears.

Where religion is a name and thus a norm, a further implication follows: the ability to understand religion is rooted in a scholar's own *experience* as well as in her rational capacity. In so far as "religion" itself is a name for a kind of experience, a phenomenologist studying religion is working with her experience of another's experience. As van der Leeuw describes:

> By "experience" is implied an actually subsisting life which, with respect to its meaning, constitutes a unity. Experience, therefore, is not pure "life," since in the first place it is objectively conditioned, and secondly, it is inseparably connected with its interpretation as experience. "Life" itself is incomprehensible. . . . For the "primal experience," upon which our experiences are grounded, has always passed irrevocably away by the time our attention is directed to it. (REM 671)

Any scholar's experience of some moment as "religion" constitutes a "unity" in the sense that it is a "third thing" as described above. As this third thing, it is informed or "objectively conditioned" by a person's concept of what religion is as developed over the range of her past experiences. As van der Leeuw notes in Schleiermachian tones, the so-called "primal experience" upon which a scholar's experience of the phenomenon is based has always "passed irrevocably away."

Van der Leeuw summarizes: "Our experience [of religion] is never a primal experience of the object itself, nor is it merely a re-experiencing of it, but it is another, relatively independent experience, which forms itself in us on account of 'signs'—e.g., words of a person, the letters of a document, the remnants of an ancient settlement—as a meaningful whole."[1] The implication for a phenomenologist seeking to understand religion then, is that the task involves cultivating an ability to recreate his own experience of *another human's experience* in order to discern whether it has meaning for that other person as what the phenomenologist recognizes as "religion." "Religion" thus takes shape as an imaginative schema, one that arises in an ongoing, open-ended dialectic between a scholar's acts of rational reflection and his experiences of meaning in relation to the chaotic maze of reality. Van der Leeuw intends his phenomenology of religion to guide scholars in courting and recreating the appearance of such imaginative schemes.

WHOSE ESSENCE?

Before turning to flesh out van der Leeuw's phenomenological method, a word is necessary to those who critique his discussions of essence as evidence of his (theological) belief in the existence of a Sacred, an entity inaccessible to scientific study. This critique of van der Leeuw represents a misreading funded by fidelity to an emergence narrative of the field.

Admittedly, the term looms large in van der Leeuw's work. As noted, however, his intent in engaging the term is to call "essentialist" appeals to essence into question. When van der Leeuw uses the term in relation to a *phenomenon*, he is not referring to a foundation or ground that is inaccessible to reason. Rather, the essence of a phenomenon *is* its appearance—that is, that set of characteristics that catches a scholar's attention and stirs her recognition of it as, in this case, religion. The essence of religion is the fabric of particulars within which a researcher finds herself suspended in the instant that something appears to her as having meaning as religion. As a fabric of particulars, essence is irreducibly relational and thus, temporal, contextual, and evolving; it bears no direct, empirical, or logical relation to historical religions or to their espoused truths; it represents an ideal type, an imaginative and organizing net of experiences that opens and forecloses further appearances of meaning. It has no reality (SRA 406). While "essence" does enjoy a certain normative transcendence over the particulars whose emergence it enables, that transcendence is, at the same time, a function of any one particular phenomenon's appearing. Any claim to an essence thus represents a conceptual web tossed over the given, concealing the actual reality of particulars even as it makes them intelligible as religion.

Further, by designating the essence of religion as an appearance, van der Leeuw displaces the distinction between a rationally defensible essence and experiential manifestations so often employed—as seen in Chapters 1 through 4—to frame "theology" as the enemy of a free-reason, theorizing religion. If "theology" errs by mistaking the phenomenal forms of a given tradition for its essence (as Kant and Schleiermacher in particular develop), then van der Leeuw's depiction of the essence as itself a manifestation challenges the terms of that exclusion in ways similar to Hegel. Any appeal to a rationally defensible essence of religion as a means for evaluating the forms of religion itself represents one more *phenomenal form* in which religion appears as having meaning. It represents a scholar reflecting upon his own experience—in this case, an experience enabled by a particular sense of the relationship between reason and experience. In sum, if a concept of essence is only one more manifestation, then the act of taking that essence for a real thing is a mistake made in "bad" theology. By fixing one expression of "religion" as definitive, a scholar arrests the self-correcting dialectic of reason and experience internal to the vitality of the phenomenon itself. He energizes only one dimension of the dialectic between reason and experience, privileging one form over the other.

If van der Leeuw had argued that essences or names captured actual reality, then it would follow that scholars in the study of religion could free their work from theology, because scholars could verify that their conceptions of the essence of religion were really true. However, where religion is a phenomenon and where the value of the term "religion" rests in its potential for rendering life intelligible, then the study of religion itself is a process of continually renegotiating the definition of religion. Scholars can secure freedom in relation to theology only by realizing that there are no grounds for opposing it other than those found in an ongoing contestation with it. Rather than reifying religion as beyond science, van der Leeuw's talk of essences points towards an understanding of objectivity that is not bound by a fixed notion of rationality.

A PRACTICE OF UNDERSTANDING

If a phenomenon is a network of relations, both created and received, equally "mine" and "its," a particular and a fabric of particulars, neither historical fact nor a tradition's doctrine, suspended amidst a plurality of experiences, then what is a person who is interested in studying religion to do? How do scholars pursue religion? How do they advance their goal of understanding the conditions of an appearance of religion? By what means do people become phenomenologists? And why does van der Leeuw persist in describing his method for understanding the phenomena of religion as *indirect*?

The number of pages van der Leeuw spends elucidating his indirect method is relatively small and concentrated in an "Epilogomena" tacked to the end of his lengthy *Religion in Essence and Manifestation.*[2] In brief, where a phenomenon is what appears, where what appears is an experience of meaning, and where the task of the phenomenologist is to recreate the conditions of that appearance, no direct approach is possible. Any attempt to analyze a phenomenon by way of a general method or formula would repress the distinctive features of an object's appearing: that is, the relationship between scholar and phenomenon. The task of phenomenologists, then, must be to cultivate vulnerability to moments in which religion "dawns upon me" as the meaning of some phenomenon: they need to develop a sensitivity in experiencing phenomena as religion, an ability to discern the structural relations enabling that appearance, and a facility in critiquing and refining the ideal types they represent so as to further deepen their openness to further appearances. In other words, phenomenologists must cultivate the ability to move both ways along a dialectic of reason and experience. Van der Leeuw's phenomenology of religion is best described as a *practice of understanding*.[3]

Specifically, van der Leeuw holds every phenomenologist responsible for practicing three interlocking capabilities: imaginative empathy, a suspension of intellectual judgment, and a willingness to move between chaos and form. A phenomenologist practices these three capabilities as the sources and standards of understanding. As we will see, it is a method uniquely matched to the kind of phenomenon that its use reveals religion to be. It is also uniquely qualified to appreciate dance as a medium of religious experience and expression.

Imaginative Empathy

The key to van der Leeuw's phenomenological practice is imaginative empathy. "Empathy" (*Einfühlung*) is a term he borrows from his reading of structural psychologists such as Dilthey, Jaspers, and Spranger, and shades with allusions to Schleiermacher, Hegel, and Kierkegaard.[4] As van der Leeuw explains, empathy refers to a person's ability to "interpolate" the experience of another into the matrices comprising her own life by "transposing" herself into the experience as it appears to her (SRA 402-3). In the case of religion, the phenomenologist seeks to recreate for herself the meaning that a given sign, whether icon, action, or belief, has for someone (a practitioner) such that it appears to her (the phenomenologist) as religion. To investigate this appearance, the phenomenologist empathizes with the practitioner by imagining what it must be like to be that human being. Her imaginative empathy engages a double movement: "transposing," a phenomenologist surrenders her own experience to draw closer to the shape of another's experience; "interpolating," she mobilizes the reaches of her own experience in order to become a network of particulars capable of helping her match (her perception of) the movement of that other's experience. It is in this double movement, according to van der Leeuw, that understanding emerges. A scholar is able to name the particular as having meaning for her in terms of an ideal type defined by a nexus of structural relations. When expressed, in turn, such understanding provides others with access to a human experience that might otherwise have appeared to them as illusory, primitive, or, in a word, incomprehensible.

In an early essay, van der Leeuw elucidates the double movement involved in imaginative empathy by comparing it to the art of swimming; here he engages the work of William James, who refers to experience as a stream of consciousness. Van der Leeuw writes:

> He who wants to experience the stream [of another human's experience] in its living coolness must learn how to swim. But this too is an art. It is not true that anyone who is not altogether stupid and who has open eyes, might become an "empathetic" psychologist. This psychological method must be learnt, and with considerable effort. Here the *phenomenological analyst* makes his appearance. (SRA 402)

To experience the "living coolness" of someone else's experience, a phenomenologist must first jump in. He must practice putting himself inside the thoughts and feelings and lived awareness of another person who appears to be doing religion. As noted above, as a phenomenologist jumps in to whatever signs of that experience remain he does not become the stream, he learns to swim in it—with it. Reaching into the depths of his own experiences, he finds and creates movements within his body that allow him to move with his perception of the stream's currents. He forms in himself an image of his movements—a structural relation. Empathy is an art. What he experiences while swimming, then, is how the act of jumping into the stream changes him—pulls, organizes, and mobilizes his own sensory past and present. By plunging in, he generates his own independent experience of what appeared to him initially as meaning religion for someone.

Then the phenomenologist reflects upon that experience of imagining herself in the stream of another's experience. The practice of imaginative empathy extends to reflecting upon this experience of swimming. In writing about her experience, a scholar recreates in words a verbal image of her own swimming movements. She expresses those elements of the stream that appeared to her while swimming as defining its character—its meaning for her as religion. In other words, in imaginative empathy, a scholar seeks to deepen and recreate her experience of another's experience by actively exercising the generative tension back and forth between her self and her perception of the other, her experiences of a phenomenon and her reflections upon those experiences. Any name she grants to a phenomenon represents her imaginative and empathetic capacity as awakened and exercised by the so-named stream.

In his definition of imaginative empathy, then, van der Leeuw seals his critique of method-driven approaches to the study of religion, regardless of whether the method is historical, social scientific, or theological. In practicing imaginative empathy, a phenomenologist is conscious of theories and methods but only in so far as they represent formative moments of the phenomenologist's own experience that a particular appearance pulls into view as the condition for its appearing. Their value must always be tested in relation to the ongoing appearances of related phenomena. Theories of religion and methods for approaching religion do serve an important function. They alert, orient, and sensitize a phenomenologist's roving gaze.[5]

However, theory and method fail when scholars rely on them to enforce a distance between researcher and phenomenon in the interest of producing "objective" scholarship. While a critical distance is "indispensable" for the process of reflection, without the complementary intimacy—the effort made to jump in and swim—a scholar will not be able to understand *religion* as a *phenomenon*. A scholar will lose the ability to affirm a phenomenon as having meaning for someone. As van der Leeuw admonishes, the relationship between researcher and phenomenon needs to "be brought into close, even the closest proximity. The distance which is indispensable to any research must not degenerate into heterogeneity. In other words, the life that is being examined should acquire its place in the life of the student himself who should understand it out of his inner self" (SRA 400-1). A method-driven approach denies the relevance of that meaning-for-me as integral to understanding why the phenomenon is religion.

In so far as religion is a phenomenon, understanding out of one's "inner self" is an indispensable condition for knowledge. An appearance must appear to someone and, as van der Leeuw avers, nothing appears to a person who is not willing to open to experience a gifting of meaning. In short, what impels a phenomenologist to recreate what appears to her can not be a quest for truth or facts per se, but a living devotion to human experience—including and especially her own (SRA 402-3). He summarizes:

> We can do no otherwise. "Reality" is always my reality . . . we must recall that everything that appears to us does not submit itself directly and immediately, but only as a symbol of some meaning to be interpreted by us . . . And this interpretation is impossible unless we experience the appearance . . . not involuntarily and semi-consciously, but intentionally and methodically . . .

It is in fact the primal and primitively human art of the actor which is indispensable to all arts, but to the sciences of the mind also:—to sympathize keenly and closely with experience other than one's own, but also with one's own experience of yesterday, already become strange! (REM 674-5)

To empathize imaginatively, a phenomenologist must maintain a constant creative oscillation between the historical, philological, archeological details of another person's experience, her experience of that experience, and her own experiences—none of which are directly present in any moment, and all of which must be remembered and reconstructed. In naming an appearance, she avoids "pure art or empty fantasy" because her imaginative recreation remains accountable to her concrete encounters with the phenomena—encounters that occasion her attempts to re-experience and recreate their appearances (REM 677). As van der Leeuw explains, for one who practices living in this oscillation between reason-informed experience and experience-enabled reflection, understanding of human acts and utterances will dawn, "unless he who comprehends has acquired too much of the professor and retained too little of the man!" (REM 675).

Epoche: the Suspension of Intellectual Judgment

Practical help for a scholar in negotiating this intimate distance is given in the second capability that a phenomenologist must practice: the suspension of intellectual judgment. Despite its central role, imaginative empathy alone does not make a phenomenologist. The ability to empathize in ways which yield phenomenological understanding also requires what van der Leeuw calls—with allusions to Husserl—the "*epoche* [sic]."[6] As early as 1926, van der Leeuw admits that empathy requires "intellectual restraint": phenomenologists must learn to suspend their inclination to question the truth or reality of the experiences that appear to them as religion. To judge a phenomenon as true (or not) prior to the work of imaginative empathy arrests the double movement required for understanding.

On the one hand, the problem is obvious: judgment, like an over-belief in method, can block the willingness of a scholar to jump in and swim, reinforcing a rigid distance between scholar and phenomenon. On the other hand, ironically enough, intellectual judgment collapses the distance between researcher and phenomenon. In either case, scholars commit a blunder which thinkers in earlier chapters would fault as "theological": they fail to preserve the distinction and proper relationship between reason and experience.

It is this second instance that is more pernicious. To judge a phe-nomenon based on an imported criterion of truth assumes that the meaning of the phenomenon lies in a claim to truth. Consequently, regardless of whether a phenomenologist judges a phenomenon as true or false, the mere intention to judge casts him as participating in the meaning he perceives the phenomenon to represent—claiming truth. The inclination to judge thus demonstrates an insufficient detachment from the phenomenon. He cannot step back to imagine why the phenomenon appears to him as a claim to truth in the first place. Fused to the phenomenon by his judgment of it, he loses his willingness and his ability to synchronize his movements with those of the phenomenon; consequently, he loses his ability to generate and recreate further experiences of its appearance to him.[7]

In this way, as van der Leeuw describes, *epoche* is not a formula to apply but an *attitude* to develop. Intellectual restraint represents a willingness to tolerate otherness, believing that any phenomenon that appears has meaning for another human being, and that that meaning is not wholly alien to one's own life: "This restraint . . . implies no mere methodological device, no cautious procedure, but the distinctive characteristic of man's whole attitude to reality" (REM 675). What a phenomenologist suspends as she develops the attitude of intellectual suspense, is *not* her "reason" per se, or her sense of self or her experience (all are critical to the imaginative enterprise), but rather the tendency to perceive the experience of another human as a challenge to her own. Only by focusing on the appearances of meaning themselves will she be able to understand what it means for someone to believe that Allah spoke to Mohammed. As an attitude towards reality, the *epoche* is "no mere methodological device" but a disposition—a willingness to try to understand rather than determine or assume whether or not a person is right. As van der Leeuw encourages, "we *know* nothing, and . . . perhaps we understand very little; but . . . to understand the Egyptian of the first dynasty is, in itself, no more difficult than to understand my nearest neighbor . . . the monuments . . . as an expression, as a human statement . . . are no harder [to understand] than my colleague's letters" (REM 676-7). Thus, as a phenomenologist develops the ability to suspend intellectual judgment, she will not necessarily enhance her knowledge of truth or history per se, but she can improve her ability to understand and represent what other humans, including her younger self, have found meaningful about truth and history.

Willingness to Move between Chaos and Form

Successful practice of imaginative empathy and intellectual suspension requires that phenomenologists develop a third capability as well: a constant willingness to suspect the adequacy of their understanding and seek new appearances of meaning that challenge its forms. The operative word here is *movement*. As van der Leeuw conveys, "all his life," the phenomenologist "oscillates hither and thither" between "the unformed chaos of the historical world and its structural endowment with form"; "the phenomenologist strides here and there" (REM 686); "the phenomenologist of religion strides backwards and forwards over the whole field of religious life" (REM 687). Where understanding is never complete, phenomenologists must repeatedly venture out from their secure world of concepts and categories and expose themselves to the rich manifold of what is given to them. They must move across cultures and languages, between historical accounts and theological evaluations, broadening their experience base, making themselves vulnerable to shocks of meaning. They must move back and forth across the fields of their own experiences as well, remembering and reassessing their potency as resources for understanding.

Such movement is critical, according to van der Leeuw, and not just for understanding. It is critical for ensuring that that understanding remains responsive to the maze of the given. In so far as religion is a phenomenon, appearing in the culturally precise relationship between researcher and the given, *movement guarantees account-ability*. Standards for objectivity arise internal to the practice of understanding, as phenomenologists actively challenge, correct, and qualify their rational reflections on their ongoing experiences of meaning. While culling insights in and through personal experiences, they avoid subjective bias by suspending intellectual judgment and practicing empathy. While making use of concepts, categories, and rational reflection, they guard against the methodological straight-jacket by constantly suspecting their conclusions and exposing them-selves to the historical record. In both directions, they avoid the charge of "theology" by preserving an open-ended dialectical tension between reason and experience. They find no ground on which to rest. As van der Leeuw puts it, "far more than all other spheres of knowledge, the phenomenology of religion is dynamic: as soon as it ceases to move it ceases to operate. Its infinite need of correction per-tains to its innermost being" (REM 695). The conscious practice of imaginative empathy, the suspension of intellectual judgment, and the need for "infinite correction" open within a human a capacity to sustain insights into what is "essential, typical and meaningful" about religion (SRA 405).

Further, phenomenologists must practice one other kind of move-ment. For phenomenologists to understand the "essence" of a reli-gious phenomenon—that is, why something appears to them as bearing meaning as religion—they must move back and forth across the boundaries of their own self-understanding, challenging their memories of their own experiences and previous insights. As phenomenologists generate new experiences for themselves and reflect upon them, they will alter their ability to experience further appearances of religious meaning. Each phenomenologist is an ever-evolving matrix of responsivity on which she or he draws in attempts to experience and interpret appearances of meaning. Or, as van der Leeuw phrases it, a phenomenologist's "understanding is identical with his being in the world."[8] As she practices imaginative empathy, the *epoche*, and movement, whatever understanding a scholar gleans will transform her. Conversely, only by practicing being open to such transformation will a person retain the flexibility to grasp new appearances as they erupt arbitrarily and unpredictably.

In so far as understanding is identical with "being in the world," van der Leeuw's phenomenologist practices doing what human beings do every day as they conduct their relations with other humans. Phenomenology is not the provenance of sequestered scholars. It cultivates a constitutive activity of human life. As van der Leeuw writes, phenomenology

> is not a method that has been reflectively elaborated, but is man's true, vital activity, consisting in losing himself neither in things nor in the *ego*, neither in hovering above objects like a god nor dealing with them like an animal, but in doing what is given to neither animal nor god: standing aside and understanding what appears into view. (REM 676)

The difference between phenomenological and "ordinary" understanding is one of intention and degree: "What matters . . . is that what is done here [in ordinary usage] unconsciously and frequently also in an entirely arbitrary manner, should receive a methodological character by means of psychological self-education" (SRA 406). Here, learning about one's *self* is not the goal but rather a means for entering into richer relations with the experiences of other humans as they appear to us and allowing ourselves to be transformed by them. The conceptual nets a scholar produces do not and cannot represent the totality of the given or of one's self and still enable meaning to appear; something must disappear, as the background of the appearing. To interrogate this selection process as it operates in the study of religion across its subfields is the work of a phenomenologist.

Acknowledging his debt to Kierkegaard, van der Leeuw compares the work of his phenomenologist to that of Kierkegaard's "psychological observer," quoting him, "not as a rule, and not even as an idea, but as a permanent reproach":

> "Just as the psychological investigator must possess a greater suppleness than a tight-rope walker, so that he can install himself within men's minds and imitate their dispositions: just as his taciturnity during periods of intimacy must be to some degree seductive and passionate, so that reserve can enjoy stealing forth ... so he must have a poetic originality within his soul, so as to be able to construct totality and orderliness from what is presented by the *individuum* only in a condition of dismemberment and irregularity."[9]

In German a tightrope walker is a dancer, a "rope dancer," *Seiltanzer*.

EMBODIED UNDERSTANDING

Van der Leeuw's commitment to the phenomenology of religion as a practice of imaginative empathy, intellectual restraint, and ceaseless movement between reason and experience, chaos and form, has repercussions for considering dance as religion at every point in the exclusionary logic documented in Chapters 1 through 4. At the most basic level, by identifying religion as a phenomenon, van der Leeuw denies any and all theories of religion—including those that function to marginalize dance—as the definitive word on religion. At the same time, not only does his work suggest that theories of religion can and do evolve, it offers guidance on how such change progresses, and in particular, how the phenomenologist participates in that development. In so far as religion represents a fabric of particulars, then phenomenologists invariably stretch and pull that fabric in response to and in order to account for phenomena that appear to them as religion. It is not just that religion exists as a category which scholars then apply to various phenomena; but rather that religion represents a net of previously experienced and recreated particulars such that each application of the term alters the definition, even if only slightly, and enables new experiences. In fact, van der Leeuw's analysis suggests, the study of religion exists as this process of defining and redefining the object it purports to study. Although there is no object per se, the exercise of defining and applying the term "religion" is nonetheless necessary because the act of doing so allows certain dimensions of human experience to register that are not accessible to empirical, logical, or quantitative analysis—namely, questions of meaning and of how humans enter into and embrace that meaning as their own. The *essence* of *religion* does elude rational explication but not because that essence is a supernatural Other. Rather, "religion" is something that appears as a meaningful phenomenon (name, ideal, type, and structure) only by virtue of a scholar's conscious study of the forms of other humans' experience and expressions. There is no reason to exclude dance per se as such a form.

Appreciating the dynamism and flexibility implied by identifying religion as a phenomenon is not in itself sufficient to ensure that the field can or will evolve to take account of dance as religion. Equally as important is the way in which van der Leeuw describes that dynamism as driven by an open-ended dialectical tension between reason and experience. A dialectic is not a balance: there is no midpoint of equal contribution. Rather, the dialectic describes an oscillation between moments in which a scholar exercises reason over experience and others in which she cultivates her vulnerability to certain kinds of experience. Neither reach of the swing is "pure": as she moves in one direction, tension with the other pole of her understanding pulls her back. A phenomenologist exercises her reason in relation to the *appearances* of meaning—not the truth of the metaphysical claims; her rational reflection is mediated and informed by those experiences. Alternately, she cultivates an experience of those *appearances*—and not of Buddha or God or the Sacred itself. Her "experience" represents a conscious submersion in an imaginative recreation of another's experience mediated by her intention to understand the categories and concepts available to her. Her "reason" remains accountable to the pull of sensory claims. In this way, van der Leeuw insists, the circularity between definition and method opens to a spiraling interplay in and through the practice of the phenomenologist.

For van der Leeuw, then, the criteria for any objective theory, method, or account of religion exist in the context of the community of people brought into being by the phenomenologist's role as a braiding, mediating thread, drawing social scientist, humanist, and theologian, scholar and practitioner, to contribute to the process of weaving wider, thicker nets of understanding, and ever testing their assumptions. It is the community constituted by all those who participate in the cultural uses and definition of religion.[10] Any attempt to study religion which presumes the possibility of clearly distinguishing between method and object, van der Leeuw would protest, misconceives the process of human understanding, the nature of "religion," and the tactics required to study it. By implication, any scholars who would deny theology a corrective and constitutive role in the project of understanding religion would weaken their own claims to objectivity.

Implicit within this vision of the phenomenology of religion is a dance-friendly implication whose repercussions for the study of religion in general, and the study of dance in particular, have yet to be developed beyond van der Leeuw's work (see Chapters 7 through 9). Understanding is a fully embodied event. Even when writing about jumping into streams of another's experience, van der Leeuw does not advocate participating directly in religious ceremonies and practices. Though an historian of religions, he rarely traveled beyond the borders of his homeland; many of the religions he studied were dead. More often than not, he was working with mere fragments of a time and place. His imaginative empathy was imaginative—a mental action, nourished by practices of reading and writing. Even so, van der Leeuw urged scholars to cultivate a dynamic dialectic between rational reflection and experiences of meaning by engaging the "life complexity" that they themselves are as the primary source and site for understanding. Van der Leeuw writes:

> In the act of understanding not merely a free and as it were transcendent consciousness is active, an observing and calculating intellect, but man's *life*, i.e., his whole existence as it expresses itself in the first place in his body, but then also in the world, in so far as he makes this world his own world. . . . A "human being" is not merely an abstract "consciousness" and even less an active intellect, but a life complexity. (OU 409)

A scholar's ability to understand religion is informed by how he lives his life. Where he orients his gaze, how he focuses his intentions, what range of experience he has available to call upon—all fund and inform his ability to receive appearances of meaning—regardless of whether a scholar actually participates in a ritual or studies textual accounts of it. The process is the same. Bound to whatever appears, a phenomenologist necessarily engages in a constant dialectical movement, producing his own capacity for a richer experience of religion's meaning as well as books, articles, and courses. In this way, van der Leeuw's phenomenology opens avenues for arguing that phenomenologists should engage in the kinds of activity that cultivate embodied experience or physical consciousness. If a human's *life* is active in understanding, then a way is open to embracing dance (along with other arts) as a practice for developing awareness of how our bodily being enables and informs our rational and experiential capacities.

Finally, Van der Leeuw's embrace of embodied understanding yields a concept of objectivity that does not depend upon an opposition to "theology." Where religion is a phenomenon, there is no possible ground in either reason or experience, in either objective method or the voice of a particular religious moment, outside of their mutual self-correcting interplay, for establishing scientific credibility. Said otherwise, the objectivity relevant for an embodied, relational understanding is internal to the dynamic of self-correction involved in a phenomenologist's practice of empathy, restraint, and movement. As van der Leeuw insists, abstraction without close attention to detail of religion produces weak categories; close attention to detail without self-conscious reflection on the larger contexts of human life (including one's own) that enable the isolation and identification of particular "religions" risks seeing only those "facts" that mirror the scholar's own theological presuppositions. Here, van der Leeuw would agree with his critics: in so far as a phenomenologist studies religion without an awareness of her mediating role between historical study and theology, she runs the risk of collapsing into one or the other—that is, into both. Conversely, to the extent that she keeps moving between facts and truths, a phenomenologist resists presenting her findings as a last word. To the extent that she keeps moving, she is able to find within herself the resources for imaginative recreation of new experiences of meaning as they continue to appear to her. Her challenge is to cultivate a generative tension in her own work, and among members of the field, so that each disciplinary perspective may come to acknowledge its responsibility in relation to the others.

The key to this objectivity lies in the three interlocking activities comprising the phenomenology of religion that impel the phenomenologist in her braiding movement between theological and social scientific or humanist approaches to the study of religion. As a phenomenologist practices his conceptual exercises, he engages and enables the work of historians. He steeps himself in the details of what happened as recorded through historical and social scientific methods; he interrogates why these details and not others appear as religion, and helps the historian assess the parameters of her thinking. Alternately, the phenomenologist listens attentively to the claims made by theologians and practitioners about the meaning of those artifacts and details as reported by and for those involved; he affirms the existence of those meanings without evaluating their merits. As he moves between these disciplines, then, a phenomenologist observes the connections forming in his mind, patterns of relation, similarity and difference. He hazards the "intoxication" of naming, and the names he generates facilitate efforts by historians and theologians in their observation, interpretation, and evaluation of human life. As van der Leeuw affirms, learning this mediating "role" is the goal of the phenomenologist of religion: "Only the persistent and strenuous application of this intense sympathy, only the uninterrupted learning of his role, qualifies the phenomenologist to interpret appearances."[11]

Van der Leeuw is well aware that the kind of objectivity that results from such a process of mutual critique and correction will not appear in the form of a convergence of ideas. In so far as phenomenologists proceed by engaging their own experiences as the source of understanding, scholars practicing this method may produce infinite interpretations regarding what causes some one thing to appear to someone as religious. Van der Leeuw would disagree, however, that such divergence disqualifies his method as "unscientific." Rather, divergence represents a sign of health—a sign of the range of resources, experiences, and perspectives that scholars are bringing to bear on questions of religion. When welcomed and cultivated, such divergence allows for a richer context of mutual critique and correction. By espousing generative tension rather than convergence, members in the field of religious studies who adopt different approaches can come to appreciate those differences as enabling each other to produce better work, whether it is in the shape of historical accounts or interpretations, theological assessments, or phenomenological understandings. As van der

Leeuw insists, "no single cognitive process is a net embracing all and everything. Science is never absolute" (OU 411).

Van der Leeuw's vision of phenomenology as a mediating thread in a braided methodological approach to religious studies gestures beyond antitheology polemics towards an ethic of contested interdependence. By animating the dialectic of reason and experience as the source of embodied understanding, and locating the locus of objectivity within the community of people a phenomenologist's braiding action brings into being, van der Leeuw defuses the fear of "theology" that drives scholars to rely on the practice of writing (as enacting the freedom of reason in relation to experience) as a guard against theology. He does so, in part, by offering an explanation, with allusion to Kierkegaard, of why such a strategy ultimately fails. When writing becomes the sole model and matrix for objective study, attachment to it arrests the movement between reason and experience crucial for a self-correcting understanding. A person or community attached to writing as the model and structure for knowledge inevitably makes a "theological" mistake: privileging either the capacity of reason to detach from and reflect upon the contents and conditions of experience or an irreducible quality of experience inaccessible to writing that eludes rational explication. Scholars privilege the ability of reason to overcome the distinction between reason and experience (as in Hegel) or rest with conviction that the gap between reason and experience enabled by reason is irreconcilable (as in Kierkegaard). By relying on the practice of writing to secure objectivity, scholars in the field fuel the hostility to theology they intend to relieve. In so doing, they divert their attention from those aspects of the given that do not conform to the way in which writing is used. As the following chapters illustrate, to take religion seriously as a phenomenon is to discern a space between theological evaluation and historical fact where a scholar may gradually develop an understanding of dancing, of rhythmic bodily movement, as object and model for the practice and products of religious study.

CHAPTER 7

Understanding Religion and Dance

> For those who do not view religion as a kind of pious entertainment, but as the daily bread of the believer—as his constant confrontation with the powers [*de Machten*] which rule all life—it is obvious that even the approach to God or to the gods can, indeed must be a dance.
>
> — Gerardus van der Leeuw, *Sacred and Profane Beauty: The Holy in Art*

There is evidence in van der Leeuw's descriptions of the phenomenological method and in his accounts of dance that it was his interest in dance, at least in part, that impelled him to design a theory of religion and a phenomenological method for the study of it that would prove flexible enough to comprehend both historical appearances of dance in world religions and theological condemnations of dance as hostile to religion. Why van der Leeuw was interested in dance and religion is difficult to determine. His interest may have been stirred by his study of Egyptian and Greek religions. The pyramid texts he analyzed for his dissertation, for example, include descriptions of dance. He may have been struck by the admonitions to dance in the Hebrew Bible. An avid musician, he also adored Bach, whose song forms are often derived from dances; he played the organ in class for his students. Conversely, he may have attended a concert performed by Isadora Duncan, the American pioneer of modern dance, a sensation in Europe, who toured the Netherlands several times.[1] He would not have found support for such interest among the members of his Dutch Reformed congregation.[2]

Regardless of its source, van der Leeuw's interest in dance appears throughout his career, evolving in tandem with his braided approach to studying religion. As early as 1930 he published an essay in Dutch and soon thereafter in German, with the title, *'In den hemel is enen dance'*.[3] He incorporated this essay into the first edition of his classic on religion and the arts, published in 1932 under the title *Wegen en Grenzen*, or "Paths and Boundaries." It was one year later that he published his 700-page manifesto for the phenomenology of religion, *Religion in Essence and Manifestation*. This sequence alone suggests that van der Leeuw was working out his phenomenological method and his reflections on religion and the arts simultaneously. Subsequently, after more than a decade of researching, employing, and teaching the history of religions, theology, and his phenomenological method, van der Leeuw substantially reworked *Wegen en Grenzen*, publishing the new edition in 1948, two years before his death. In the same year he published his *Sacramentstheologie*. In this second edition of *Wegen en Grenzen*, dance assumes a more prominent role than earlier, appearing as the first of six arts whose relationship to religion he explores.[4] Van der Leeuw even makes a case for why dance provides the paradigm for thinking about the relation of every other art to religion in general, and to Christianity in particular.

How, then, does van der Leeuw's braided approach to the study of religion and his theory of religion as a phenomenon support his willingness and ability to acknowledge dance as religion? The first step in answering this question is to lay out the definition of religion his phenomenological method guides him to generate, and then, in the latter part of this chapter and the two following, explore how this conceptual net guides him in acknowledging and making sense of historical and theological accounts of religion.

What is religion? In the "Epilegomena" as well as in the body of *Religion in Essence and Manifestation,* van der Leeuw hazards his own perspectives on the "essence" of religion (as qualified above) based on his years of practicing phenomenology, moving across the landscape of human history, between historical studies and theological evaluations, between the manifold chaos of the given and the structural relations he evolves to net instances of religion. Simply, a phenomenon appears to him as religion when it appears as an expression of *power*.[5] A text, icon, activity, art object, architectural design, musical composition, or other "sign" appears as religion in so far as it appears to congeal, conduct, catalyze, or concentrate an experience of change in human thought and/or action.[6] Van der Leeuw's dynamic method produces a dynamic definition.

The kind of power whose expression appears as religion is one that occurs at the intersection of what van der Leeuw calls two "planes" of life: horizontal and vertical. First, power appears in the form of human agency. All shapes of culture humans use or manufacture— whether linguistic, artistic, economic, or political—express power in this sense. They express the capacity and the inclination people have to create the world in which they desire to live. As van der Leeuw writes, a person seeking power "tries to elevate life, to enhance its value, to gain for it some deeper and wider meaning" (REM 679). He continues: "Over the variety of the given he throws his systematically fashioned net on which various designs appear: a work of art, a custom, an economy . . . and thus he develops power . . . he never halts" (REM 679). Striving to encompass greater swaths of life within their circles of experience, understanding, and control, people arrange the pieces available to them into "significant wholes" capable of guiding more comprehensive insight and action such that their living becomes more real or vivid. In this sense, power, prefiguring Foucault, is a function of knowledge—who has it, who can use it, who benefits from it, and who determines what qualifies as it.[7] Power is the ability to establish as dominant one's vision of the way things are. As such, power is both means and end; people exercise their power in seeking power as a potential for making "life." As humans exercise what they are given in creating and acquiring more, they map a horizontal plane of human existence.

Not all forms of human culture, however, bear the distinguishing marks of religion. Those that appear as religion are those that lay claim to the horizon within which human life has meaning, "the extension of life to its uttermost limit" (REM 680). As van der Leeuw writes, "the religious significance of things . . . is that on which no wider nor deeper meaning whatever can follow. It is the meaning of the whole: it is the last word" (REM 680). Texts, artifacts, and actions that delimit the horizon of meaning are those that appear within a culture as claiming explanatory and normative authority over all other forms of culture. They appear to represent the ends and edges of life: birth and death; purpose, meaning, and values; the furthest reach of any sensory, intellectual, emotional, or physical capability. In this sense, religion appears as the farthest flung nets humans cast in their attempts to enhance and elevate themselves and their worlds.

In laying claim to the horizon of meaning, those phenomena appearing as religion also evoke a vertical plane of power: such phenomena express human agency on the horizontal plane as a function of being or having been transected by some source of power other than human agency, a power which lies beyond the horizon of human knowing and doing. Van der Leeuw describes such "vertical" eruptions thus:

> Man, seeking power in life, does not reach the frontier; but he realizes that he has been removed to some foreign region . . . [He] knows quite definitely that *something meets him on the*

road. It may be the angel who goes before him and will lead him safely: it may be the angel with the flashing sword who forbids him the road. But it is quite certain that something foreign has traversed the way of his own powerfulness . . . this strange element has no name whatever . . . [and] can be approached only *per viam negationis*. (REM 681)

In pursuit of power-knowledge, people find themselves transported unexpectedly—resisted or empowered, guided or confused—in ways which do not correspond in a causal or logical manner to the strength of their actions and intentions. The sensation of "something foreign" crossing the path of their own agency is undeniable. What is usual, familiar, and expected appears disrupted and dislocated (REM 23). Yet nothing appears—no object or being, nothing to experience, nothing to name, nothing on which to reflect. This dislocating "angel" may (not) appear at any point on the horizontal plane. When it does, humans respond by representing this experience in terms of a power whose absence they suffer—as "a revelation, which never becomes completely experienced, though it participates in experience" (REM 680). Van der Leeuw continues, "We can never comprehend God's utterance by means of any purely intellectual capacity: what we can understand is only our own answer; and in this sense too, it is true that we have the treasure only in an earthen vessel" (REM 680-1). Religion as an expression of power appears in the forms of lines, traces of what can be imagined as vertical planes, intersecting at the horizon, connecting humans to what must always lie beyond the horizon, inaccessible to both their experience and their rational reflection upon it. Humans make, validate, and honor earthen vessels—doctrines, beliefs, practices, norms, values—which register the implications of uncanny eruptions in terms of the implications for human horizons. In so doing, people claim to provide circles of meaning within which all particular forms of life derive their purpose—as a function of something they cannot know.

Van der Leeuw concludes that it is this double character of power—agential and dislocating, horizontal and vertical—that gives phenomena that appear as religion their distinguishing quality. Such phenomena appear as self-contradictory. They participate in what van der Leeuw calls a *paradox of revelation and concealment*. As he explains, any "last word" is "never understood" and "never spoken": it is "a secret which reveals itself repeatedly, only nevertheless to remain eternally concealed . . . . the ultimate meaning is at the same moment the limit of meaning" (REM 680). A horizon cannot be made present. With every attempt to reach a horizon, it recedes. Its parameters shift in relation to a person's actions and orientation. In other words, a last word has meaning as "last" only when it is not—that is, only when humans hear it, grasp its appearance in the webs of their own understanding, and alter their action in accord with the horizon of possibility it defines.

Surveying human history, van der Leeuw observes time and again instances where humans exercise their agency by drawing horizons that represent human power as dislocated by uncanny eruptions deriving from elsewhere. Such expressions of power reveal human preoccupation with the inevitable and unavoidable presence (that is, absence) of an enabling beyond that is always already concealed from view.

Employing his phenomenological method, then, van der Leeuw produces a definition of religion that is at once comparative and contextual. A phenomenon appears as religion in so far as it demonstrates 1) a privileged status (as a "last word") in relation to other elements in the cultural context of which it is one moment, and 2) where that privilege manifests in the form of a paradox—concealing what it purports to reveal, or revealing something as always already absent. His definition of religion does not posit a universal "essence" that is either rational (as in Kant) or experiential (as in Schleiermacher), either the dialectical unity of reason and experience (as with Hegel's spirit) or their antithesis (as for Kierkegaard's

Silentio). By identifying the essence of religion with its appearance to someone as a paradoxical expression of power, van der Leeuw stretches his definition to include both directions of the dialectic between a scholar's "reason" and "experience": the essence of religion appears as the fruit of a scholar's ongoing effort to experience the meaning of human artifacts and reflect upon those experiences by recreating the form of phenomena in terms of a paradox of revelation and concealment. Any account of religion thus articulates the moments represented by Kierkegaard as "writing" and "dancing"— that is, moments that yield to and resist, respectively, the free play of reason over experience.

Moreover, contrary to what some of his critics allege, van der Leeuw's definition does not presuppose the existence of an Other or Sacred or universal essence as a Power lurking behind the phenomenal forms of religion. By understanding religious phenomena in terms of a paradox of revelation and concealment, van der Leeuw is able to explain the apparent inexplicability of religious claims as integral to their success: humans express and acquire power over the ends of life by naming (and thereby relating themselves to) a realm of disruptive, uncanny, enabling power which recedes beyond their farthest reach with every claim to master it. As van der Leeuw insists, the phenomenologist never departs from the horizontal plane. She never seeks to determine whether or not such a realm of disruptive power really exists. Rather, she seeks to understand what it means for people to represent their lives and selves as open to transformation by an experience of power they can neither fully experience nor represent. To this end, van der Leeuw affirms that such claims to a Sacred other or realm have meaning for people, and he seeks to understand that meaning by recreating the forms of these phenomena through acts of imaginative empathy.

With this definition, as Chapters 8 and 9 explore, van der Leeuw opens a path for appreciating and understanding *as religion* forms of human culture that *do not* reflect, justify, or realize the practice of writing. He does so, in addition, in a discussion that integrates the two faces of power often separated in contemporary discourse as the psychic and the social, the powers of creating and being created, which flow through and compose a human subject.[8]

A VICIOUS CIRCLE?

With this definition, however, van der Leeuw's work also takes a puzzling twist: his definition of religion appears to include the phenomenological method itself. When phenomenologists engage in a quest for understanding, moving back and forth between historical records and theological claims, recalling past experiences with existential situations engaged, waiting for understanding to appear, are they *religious*? Is van der Leeuw engaged here in a vicious circularity where the object "religion" is defined as that which his method can discern, such that the ability to understand appearances is always guaranteed and the use of the phenomenological method always justified?[9] Van der Leeuw demurs: a phenomenologist does participate in a paradox of revelation and concealment which "is certainly essential to all religions, but also to all understanding" (REM 683). Yet for him, this common participation is the link that resolves the problem framed by theorists read in earlier chapters—namely, how to ensure scholarship that is both objective and empathetic. For van der Leeuw, the phenomenology of religion demonstrates its difference from religion based on how it participates in this paradox. In brief, for the phenomenologist, what a given earthen vessel reveals as concealed is not "God" per se, but the meaning of *religion*.

Given that the term "religion," like all cultural creations, is a conceptual net tossed over the manifold of the given, phenomenologists do participate in the paradox of revelation and concealment, and they do so in at least two ways. First, as noted in the previous chapter, every time phenomenologists apply the term "religion," they reveal the particular they intend to represent by concealing its "actual reality"; its meaning appears as given by its relations to other particulars that appear to share the quality that renders them intelligible. As the name for a phenomenon, "religion" must conceal in order to facilitate understanding of what it reveals.

In so far as phenomenologists are aware of this dynamic and cultivate it, they participate in a second paradox of revelation and concealment. In practicing the phenomenological method, phenomenologists do exercise their agency in weaving conceptual nets, yet they simultaneously nourish their vulnerability to being surprised by something foreign. They seek to have their understanding displaced by a "revelation" of meaning that conceals differently. As van der Leeuw avers, "*all* comprehension, without exception, ultimately reaches the limit where it loses its own proper name and can only be called 'becoming understood'" (REM 683). At its limit, then, "all comprehension, irrespective of whatever object it refers to, is ultimately religious: all significance sooner or later leads to ultimate significance" (REM 684). In this way, for van der Leeuw, the practice of phenomenology itself does express power, and in a paradoxical form: phenomenologists pursue the power of understanding by continually submitting their concepts and categories to the dawning of meaning, to the moments of "becoming understood."

Nevertheless, practicing the phenomenology of religion is not religion in this sense: phenomenologists submit their understanding for correction to the historical record and theological evaluations, not to a god, Other, or process of enlightenment. More importantly, in recreating the forms in which earthen vessels appear to them, they do not pretend to offer a last word. In fact, in so far as phenomenologists participate consciously in the paradox of revelation and concealment common to understanding, they are thereby able to recognize the paradox expressed in religion and, at the same time, distinguish themselves from religion: they can affirm that people do make claims about what cannot be revealed, without themselves passing judgment on whether those claims are true. Their concern is to understand the meaning that such representations of human experience have for the humans who honor them. Van der Leeuw writes: "it is indeed precisely because it [the paradox] holds good for *both,* for religion and understanding alike, that our science becomes possible ... faith and intellectual suspense (the *epoche*) do not exclude each other" (REM 683).

Here van der Leeuw makes his case for an approach to religious studies that acknowledges an irresolvable contradictory tension between affirmative and critical moments as integral to the process of understanding religion. In so far as religion is a phenomenon, any affirmation of a particular as religion proceeds by way of a critical moment in which its particularity is concealed; any rational account of religion, in turn, proceeds by way of an affirming moment in which the phenomenon appears as having meaning for the way it eludes rational explication. Scholars who participate in this tension generate understanding that is at once objective (within the community of mutual correction brought into being by the mediating work of the phenomenologist); empathetic (in its efforts to recreate the paradoxical form of revelation and concealment in which a phenomenon appears as having meaning as religion); and dynamic (as a self-conscious expression of power). The moments of the phenomenological process cannot be reconciled without losing the intimate distance needed for understanding and collapsing into "theology" or, for that matter, "history."

TESTING A DEFINITION

So then, does it work? How does van der Leeuw's definition of religion as a paradoxical expression of power help make sense of dance as religion? His definition sports at least three advantages that I will discuss in turn. Generally speaking, the definition of religion van der Leeuw generates by way of his phenomenological method blazes the way for displacing the primary role accorded to linguistic forms as models for the objects, methods, and outcomes of studying religion.

First, where religion is a paradoxical expression of power, the phenomenologist is responsible for seeking out forms of human culture where a phenomenon appears to someone as meaningful based on its ability to articulate and make known this paradox. Such a definition of religion predisposes a phenomenologist to look for forms of culture whose meaning lies in their *resistance* to verbal translation—forms of expression that exist in a conflicted relation with writing. Correlatively, a scholar practicing van der Leeuw's phenomenological approach may be drawn to study dance practice and performance as religion in cases where dancing participates in a paradox of revelation and concealment relative to verbal forms of religion. By this logic, the quality of dance that has proved the greatest obstacle to its consideration as religion (a perceived opposition to writing) emerges as its most interesting feature.

Further, in so far as phenomenologists pursue forms of human culture that demonstrate a paradoxical form, they are constantly reminded as well of their own participation in the paradoxes of revelation and concealment common to all understanding. As such, they can no longer sustain a belief in writing as a medium for rendering the essence or meaning of religion transparent to rational thinking. Instead, they must develop an appreciation of how their commitment to writing as a mode and model of scholarship serves as an effective conduit for understanding religion *by concealing* aspects of the phenomena they intend to study. In practicing the phenomenological method, scholars develop a sense of responsibility for what the medium of their understanding conceals.

Finally, this realization is not grounds for dismissing writing. It is impossible for scholars not to conceal part of what they are trying to reveal in naming religion. Rather, van der Leeuw's definition of religion suggests that scholars need to practice a kind of activity that affords an experience of writing's limits. Such an activity would foster a scholar's ability to empathize imaginatively with forms of experience whose meaning lies in the ways in which they contest translation into verbal form and help her conceptualize and maximize the efficacy of writing in facilitating understanding. In this reading, practicing an activity such as dance might thus serve as a means for defusing the kind of positions for and against "theology" that the practice of writing appears to justify.

RELIGION AND DANCE

Van der Leeuw puts his definition of religion and its implications for acknowledging dance as a medium of religious experience and expression to the test in his classic, *Wegen en Grenzen* [*Paths and Boundaries*], known in English as *Sacred and Profane Beauty: The Holy in Art*. On first glance, the problem that van der Leeuw poses for himself in this book is purely a theological one: to explore the relationship between on one hand the arts as manifestations of human intelligence or "spirit" (*de genoemde vormen van geestesleven*), and on the other, "God's revelation in Christ [*Gods openbaring in Christus*]" (W xiv). In accomplishing this theological project, however, van der Leeuw rejects traditional theological methods and mobilizes a braided approach instead. He proposes to investigate the "paths and boundaries" that connect and separate appearances of "religion" and "art" across historical traditions, time periods, and geographical locations as the basis for reflecting upon the relation of the arts to God's revelation in Christ. Van der Leeuw's task is historical and phenomenological: he aims to recreate the forms of phenomena that pull these two conceptual nets (religion and art) into view, so as to discern the structural relations that define the coincidences of their meaning. Dance— "beautiful movement"— is one of six arts whose relation to religion he considers.

More specifically, in seeking to recreate the "essential connections" (literally, "binding of essences" [S 3; W 2]) or "comprehensible associations" between dance and religion, van der Leeuw intends to delineate the forms of phenomena which make sense (to him) as both an experience of beautiful movement and a paradox of revelation and concealment expressing power over the ends of life (S 6; W 4). Art, for van der Leeuw, is the name for an "experience of beauty": "The impression and expression of the beautiful we usually call art" (S 5-6; W 3-4). For van der Leeuw (following Kant), a person experiences beauty when he recognizes a sense of order. Beauty names a kind of experience in which the emergent form of a phenomenon—whether he is creating it or simply observing it—enables a person to receive or express a relation to a sense of pattern, and render it intelligible, even if as an open-ended mystery. When van der Leeuw identifies dance as an art, then, he is not suggesting that there is some property (such as beauty) that inheres within dance, but rather, that there are moments in history when a subject (whether artist or appreciator) experiences human motion as a conduit for an experience of beauty. Such a moment is also religion if it is perceived as conducting an experience of power. He is interested in the relationship between acts or experiences of meaning. As van der Leeuw insists: "We limit the question of the relationship between Beauty and Holiness to the analysis of the relationship between Beauty and Holiness as man experiences them; that is to say, [between] the holy act [*heilige handeling*] and the beautiful act [*schoone handeling*], or art."[10] What enables such an experience, van der Leeuw asks? Can art awaken in those who create or appreciate it a consciousness that a scholar recognizes as religion—that is, consciousness of intruding power pressing in from nowhere? He asks: "can art be a holy act?" (S 6; W 5).

In delimiting a braided methodological approach to the human experiences of coincidences between art and religion, van der Leeuw distinguishes his project from those in either philosophical or theological aesthetics. He is not concerned with whether a "wholly other" lies behind the phenomena, or whether there exists a universal structure of human cognition enabling a perception of dance or religion. He is not interested in defining Beauty or Holiness *an sich* as entities that have some reality in themselves, or in determining whether beauty is a function of "nature" or "intellect." He is not interested in categorizing the dancer as genius or prophet; or listing criteria by which dance might count as religion.[11] He seeks to understand—to experience and recreate the structural relations that allow something to appear to someone as both religion and dance. To the extent that van der Leeuw's phenomenological discussion provides categories and concepts capable of helping scholars name and comprehend such historical and theological instances of religion and dance, he demonstrates the value of his approach—its potentiality—in grasping emergent complexities of religious phenomena in context.

By engaging his phenomenological method in response to an ostensibly theological project, van der Leeuw demonstrates its value for the study of dance and religion in particular. Using his historically informed phenomenological analyses of non-Christian religious art in order to challenge Christian theological evaluations of art for the narrow phenomenological understandings they presuppose, van der Leeuw exposes the peculiar historicity of Christian assumptions about dance.[12] He challenges the legacy of those assumptions in Western culture in general, and in the theory and method of the study of religion, in particular. Thus, van der Leeuw's braided method provides him with the means to resist the ignorance of dance perpetuated by both theological and antitheological impulses within the study of religion. He produces insights with beguiling originality.

At the same time, in framing a phenomenological inquiry into coincidences of dance and religion, van der Leeuw admits that the task he is undertaking is impossible. As conceptual nets, "dance" and "religion" elicit meaning in so far as they impose meaning. They allow related things and meanings to appear only by forcing other related things and contexts to fall away. While they enable juxtaposition and comparison of varied phenomena, they are doomed to misrepresent what they claim to reveal, characterizing whole swaths of human experience through the perspective of one place and time. They are singular names where the manifold of the given is chaotically plural

(S 266; W 262-3). Invoking these names, van der Leeuw is invariably biased from the beginning by what he is able and willing to observe. He does not pretend otherwise. His response, rather, is to wield his terms as self-consciously as possible, submitting them to constant interrogation by other historians and theologians with the intent of opening up possibilities for understanding across time, space, and culture.[13] At the end of his preface, he concludes: "We are fully convinced that this [phenomenological] method has its limitations. That it is nevertheless unavoidable for all historical as well as systematic [i.e., theological] analyses we shall show by our practical experiment, rather than by theoretical disputations" (S 6; W 5).

READING *Sacred and Profane Beauty*: A CAVEAT

Before proceeding to van der Leeuw's "practical experiment," a word of warning: the project of tracing the phenomenological strands of his project is complicated by the convoluted publication history of this text. The English version represents the translation of a translation of an edition completed seven years after van der Leeuw's final revision, and five years after his death in 1950. A colleague, E. Smelik, produced the third edition, published in 1955, adding the subtitle "Reflections on the relationship between religion and art."[14] Frau Dr. Annelotte Piper translated this edition into German as *Vom Heiligen und der Kunst* ("The Holy and Art") (1957),[15] and David Green translated her German text into the English—*Sacred and Profane Beauty: The Holy in Art* (1963).[16] Along the way, the interests of editors and translators in resolving the generative tension of van der Leeuw's braided approach have at times conflicted with van der Leeuw's own.[17]

An excellent example of the difficulty in remembering the mediating role of van der Leeuw's phenomenology through the layers of the book's transmission history appears in the English title of the work: *Sacred and Profane Beauty: The Holy in Art*. The title is misleading at best. Van der Leeuw insists repeatedly in this work that any attempt to approach the relationship between religion and art through the distinction between "sacred" and "profane" fails. When scholars begin by assuming the difference between the sacred and profane, they are forced to conceive any relationship of art to religion as external to what makes the art *art*. From this perspective, the qualities that make art appear as religion are added to it; art becomes religious when it meets certain criteria accidental to its status as art— a religious content, traditional aesthetic form, context of use, etc. Van der Leeuw counters: "With an external division into 'sacred' and 'profane,' one will never achieve an expression of the holy in art. 'Holy' material is never the cause of art [*maakt geen kunst*—'does not make art'], least of all religious art" (S 268; W 441). Van der Leeuw wants to know whether there is an *internal* relationship between art and religion—whether the form that identifies an act as art may serve as a conduit for an experience of power as well. As he sees it, the term "sacred beauty" is redundant; "profane beauty" an oxymoron.

When read in light of van der Leeuw's own words, the English title is almost comical. Most likely, it was chosen to reinforce the impression of van der Leeuw as a "phenomenologist" of religion by recalling the work of another celebrated mid-century phenomenologist, Mircea Eliade, who wrote the Foreword to the English translation. Yet such an association misrepresents both van der Leeuw's phenomenology and his intent in this book. Not only is his phenomenology idiosyncratic, he did not intend this book as a pure phenomenology of religion. It is a braided work—one that consciously engages theological goals in a critical and constructive study of religion and art. In his Foreword to the 1948 edition—which does not appear in Smelik's 1955 edition or its translations into German and English—van der Leeuw explains that part of his intent in writing this *vernieuwde boek* or "renewed book" is to clarify his outline of the theological "sequel" (*verlog*) to his phenomenological studies, and thereby to draw the theological perspective into "focus" (*gezichtsveld*) such that theology may "reclaim her rights" in discussions about art. Like his theological works, Van der Leeuw wrote the text in Dutch, not in German, as he did his phenomenological treatises. The book is best represented, then, by its original title: *Paths and Boundaries.*

Given its braided composition and publication history, the challenge in reading this text is twofold: first, to resist moments in the editing and translation of the work which seek to "rescue" its phenomenological elements from theological distortion; and second, to read the relationship between its phenomenological and theological impulses as van der Leeuw intended—in two directions. As we shall see, not only does van der Leeuw's phenomenology serve his theology, but his image of what Christian revelation is—such that phenomenology may serve it—is always already informed by the structures and types which his phenomenological practice surfaces. While some critics accuse van der Leeuw of slipping among disciplines as if the work were a "game,"[18] his intertwining of history, theology, and phenomenology provides evidence of the *play* that allows van der Leeuw to avoid both the theological and antitheological obstacles to identifying dance in other cultures as internally related and critically relevant to the study of religion in general, and Christian thought and practice in particular.

In Chapters 8 and 9, as I follow the strands of this book, I read van der Leeuw's words as the play of his method demands it—on the move. In his writing, van der Leeuw moves constantly among a network of points in order to coax structural relationships between holiness and beauty into view. He slides from Christianity to and from other religions; from "religious" to and from "aesthetic"; from "primitive" to and from "modern"; between historical facts and theological claims; among artists, art objects, and appreciators; back and forth among the structural relations he defines for each art, as well as among the six arts he targets for consideration. His movement is incessant, nonlinear, and unbound by the section and heading indicators which nevertheless appear. As such, the clarity of his deceptively simple prose, once pondered, soon becomes a complex web of intercrossing associations, with each statement implicating others and shedding a different light on the guiding questions. To the words he uses—words that appear to be common enough—van der Leeuw inevitably gives a peculiar spin, deflecting complacent readings and demanding deeper reflection. Where van der Leeuw appears to give the reader a foothold, the ground invariably shifts and the reader finds herself suspended in a world whose certainties are born of faith and practice. In an attempt to keep up with van der Leeuw's kinetic methods, I leap back and forth among translations and editions, sideways to complementary passages in *Sacred and Profane Beauty* and other relevant works, and forward and backward in time to texts of other recent thinkers whose work I find helpful in apprehending van der Leeuw's play.

SEEKING "PATHS AND BOUNDARIES"

In the course of *Sacred and Profane Beauty*, Van der Leeuw's "practical experiment" unfolds as follows. For each of six arts—dance, drama, literature, visual art, architecture, music—he organizes historical cases from around the world according to five phenomenological structures, each representing possible appearances of holy acts and beautiful acts in relation to one another. They are as follows: unity of religion and art, or the "primitive"; breakup or transition to conflict; enmity between religion and art, or the "modern" of antithesis; moments of reconciliation; and finally, harmony of religion and art. He concludes each discussion with a section on "theological aesthetics" in which he distills implications that are often critical of Christian evaluations of art.

As phenomenological *structures* mapping coincidences of religion and dance, these varying configurations of identity and difference are neither chronologically nor causally related.[19] In each, van der Leeuw gathers examples from across time and culture, juxtaposing ancient traditions and his contemporary situation. In fact, van der Leeuw evokes these terms in order to resist their temporal cast.[20] As noted earlier, he laments the tendency of his colleagues to impose an evolutionary schema on the history of religions as a way to explain religious forms and their meanings. He counters that "primitive" and "modern" refer to a modern scholar's perception of reality and not reality itself.[21] He writes that

> "primitive" never means the intellectual situation of earlier times or other lands, and "modern" never that of here and now. Neither is a description of a stage in the evolution of the human spirit; rather, both are structures. We find them both realized today just as much as three thousand years ago . . . as the primitive is never completely lacking even in the most modern cities, so the modern is present in the least-educated native of Surinam [*Nieuw-Hollander*].[22]
>
> Van der Leeuw's concern is that scholars employ terms such as primitive and modern in order to defend a real difference in humanity between humans "out there" or "back then," and "us" as citizens of the "modern" world.[23] As always, he is committed to facilitating understanding among peoples—an understanding fully aware of its participation in paradoxes of revelation and concealment and its inherent incompleteness. To emphasize the provisional, perspectival, yet intellectually enabling character of such structures, van der Leeuw introduces them as *geestesstructuren*,[24] often qualifying his use of them with the phrase "so-called."
>
> In the course of van der Leeuw's experiment, dance is the first art to appear, under the heading: "Beautiful [Movement] [*De Schoone Beweging*]."[25] Among the arts in van der Leeuw's scheme, dance fills out the five phenomenological categories as no other art does; and concomitantly represents the paradigm

for art as holy act.[26] In subsequent sections of the book, the way in which a given art magnifies an element of dance defines that art's potency to conduct an experience of holiness. On the basis of these observations, van der Leeuw argues that even though dance may be lost to culture as art or religion, as long as there are arts in relation to which humans experience awe, the potential remains for dance to be reborn as an "expression of life [*een gewone levensuiting*]" (S 56; W 71). Discussing how he arrives at this conclusion requires tracing his analysis of dance through the five structures that describe possible meanings ascribed to the relationship between art and religion. Chapter 8 offers a close reading of the first of those structures, and Chapter 9, the remaining four.

Spinning the Unity of Life
Dance as Religion

The first comprehensible association van der Leeuw discusses under each art—namely, the "unity" between a given art and religion—appears most highly developed in his chapters on dance. Conversely, most of the historical examples he gives for dance fall within the rubric of this structural relation as opposed to the four discussed in Chapter 9. This pattern of distribution foreshadows van der Leeuw's conclusion that beautiful movement appears to him as "religion" or an expression of power, where it appears to express a "unity of life [*levenseenheid*]" (S 33; W 34).

As this chapter and the next will demonstrate, a claim that at first glance seems tautological—namely, that dance appears as religion where dance enacts the unity of dance and religion—harbors a radical insight into questions raised by this book. As we will see, van der Leeuw provides an explanation for why efforts in modern philosophy and theology to theorize a scientific study of religion over and against "theology" require, on phenomenological grounds, the exclusion or marginalization of dance as a medium of religious experience and expression.

This chapter progresses towards its conclusion by investigating how van der Leeuw puts the word *eenheid* or "one-ness" in spin. This term is his imaginative recreation of the form in which a phenomenon appears to him as dance and religion. When he asserts that dance *appears* as a "simple unity [*een simpele eenheid*]," he does not imply that dance *is* a simple unity. As the discussions of body and culture below elaborate, dancing *enacts*—that is, represents and brings into being as one—the complex webs of personal and communal experiences, symbolic and social relations that make the moment of performing (whether solo or in a group, alone or for a crowd) possible. For van der Leeuw, the ability of dancing to project kinetic images of unity is a primary source of its creative potency. In other words, the unity a dancer represents is a unity her movement creates *and* discloses as real in the moment of her dancing. As every dance is a unique event, so too are the unities that any act of dancing makes apparent.

Van der Leeuw is well aware that his decision to name dance as enacting a unity of life may seduce his readers into believing that dance is religious because it represents a real "Unity" existing out there apart from the dance. As the following exposition of his work attests, van der Leeuw guards against this seduction by focusing his analysis on how dancing *generates appearances* of "life" as a oneness. His point is that human dancing as beautiful movement also appears as a paradoxical expression of power as described in Chapter 7. Dancing can and does effect (*make* happen) kinetic images and experiences of "reality significantly organized" (REM 672). In doing so, dancing participates in a paradox of revelation and concealment, revealing by concealing a multiplicity of human experiences; it frames any unity it projects as an *unspeakable* "last word."

In the reading that follows, I identify two entwined arcs of "life" whose "unity" any given dance *enacts*: bodily life and cultural life. Any phenomenon that appears as dance generates kinetic images of both at once. In writing, I consider one at a time, briefly introducing van der Leeuw's comments on "the body" before elaborating those comments in the context of elucidating what he means by "culture." Along the way I tease out of van der Leeuw's work a range of concepts that will prove helpful to scholars interested in grasping the significance of rhythmic bodily life in the study of what appears to them as religion. The discussion will roam far and wide across time and space, religion and art, before returning to meditate on its implications for attempts to theorize "religion" in relation to "dance."

DANCE AS BODILY BECOMING

In laying out his phenomenological account of moments in which dance appears as both art and religion, as a conduit for simultaneous experiences of beauty and power, van der Leeuw begins with the human body. "Dance," as he defines it, is an activity that takes as its instrument the medium through which all humans live—a human body. As van der Leeuw insists, the art of dance requires nothing else for its performance other than this basic unit of life.[1] For this reason, dance may be both the oldest of the arts and the most ubiquitous: "Before man learned how to use any instruments at all, he moved the most perfect instrument of all, his body" (S 13; W 32). Van der Leeuw elaborates: Dance

> is the most universal of all the arts . . . It is an expression of all
> the emotions of the spirit, from the lowest to the highest. It
> accompanies and stimulates all the processes of life, from hunt-
> ing and farming to war and fertility, from love to death . . . To
> dance, one needs nothing, not paint, or stone, nor wood, nor
> musical instrument; nothing at all except one's own body. Man
> can produce for himself the rhythm which induces the body to
> dance (though, of course, others may do this); it is marked out
> by the stamping of feet and clapping of hands. Verbal art has
> just as little need of material or instruments, but it needs
> thought which is articulated in an image. The dance is its own
> articulation [*De dans is de articulatie zelve*]. In the greatest
> simplicity [*eenvoud*], it remains constant, century after century.
> (S 12-13; W 10-11)

In this quotation, van der Leeuw's allusions to dance as "the most universal of all the arts," expressing "all the motions" and "all the processes of life," the form that is "its own articulation" and that embodying "the greatest simplicity" all elaborate his point that dance makes apparent a unity of bodily life.

First, dance is "the most universal" of the arts because doing it requires nothing other than one's own body. Every human being *is* a body moving. Its movement is its life. A human being cannot *not* move and still live, however small these movements may be. Further, bodily movement is the medium in and through which human beings do everything that they do—think, feel, work, create, and pray.[2] A body is present in all moments of life, in all processes of life, registering the passage of time, the passing through space. Dancing, then, by displaying a body in motion, displays the medium in which all manifestations of human life—all thoughts, emotions, and actions—occur. In doing so, it connects all persons in any given society as members in and through the range of individual tasks and activities their bodies perform. The process of being and becoming body is a condition which all humans share.

At the same time, van der Leeuw is not suggesting that humans share the same body or that all bodies are the same. Even as embodiment identifies all humans as members of the same species, embodiment is also the medium that isolates every human as a radical individual. Every body is someone's body, marked by gender, race, coloring, shape, and capability. Moreover, that bodily individuality is not sui generis; its meaning as well as its development represent the unique nexus of personal, familial, social, cultural, and environmental influences any one body endures. For this reason, dance is not only "the most universal" of the arts, but also "its own articulation." Every moving human body expresses a singular crossing of personal experience and cultural formation. And that singularity extends to the moment of dancing: the meaning of any instance of dancing is inseparable from the moment in which a given individual body performs it. Following a Schleiermachian logic, then, dance is "universal" in the sense that every moment of dancing is irreducibly singular. There is no universal form or idea into which the meaning of dance can be translated. Nevertheless, what resists translation is not a sensory immediacy—not a pre-reflective, pre-verbal experience. Rather, it is the way in which dancing engages and articulates a body that is already itself a conduit of consciousness. What resists translation, with echoes of Kierkegaard, is a later immediacy—the fruits of training, practice, and discipline. Every dance appears as its own articulation, distinguished from myriad other human arts and activities, by animating the medium that they share.

Correlatively, in van der Leeuw's analysis, the "greatest simplicity" of dance appears as a function of its distinctive reflexivity.[3] In dancing, a body appears as what it is—a body—and as a *kinetic image* of itself, one stylized in movement forms: a dancer is who she is, and the image of herself that she is making in dance. A dancer is an individual articulating her individuality and a human expressing her humanity. Yet a dancer is not simply double. As she makes the movements of a dance, she changes. By moving, she develops patterns of strength and awareness. She develops a *physical consciousness*—that is, a sense of how her bodily being participates in acquiring experience and knowledge. As such, her dancing animates these discrete moments—her bodily self and kinetic images of her self—as two moments in a dialectical process of bodily becoming. In and through her dancing, she is becoming; she is also representing her ability to become, her ability to learn to make and execute movements. Said otherwise, dancing expresses a unity of bodily life by enacting a *logic of bodily becoming*—a logic particular to a body and characteristic of human bodies, which finds expression through a body's own self-doubling movement.[4]

In this reading, when van der Leeuw describes dance as "constant," that constancy appears as a function of its endless variety. Dancing describes the self-generating action of an infinite number of different bodies, female and male, young and old, bodies of various colors, ethnicities, and classes, scattered throughout space and time. Dancing appears as constant in so far as every image of unity that dancing makes apparent is kinetic, a singular, ephemeral, culturally informed expression of a body in the process of becoming. Dance thus (as described in the sections that follow) names an experience of whole- ness or order that is both grasped and lost in the moment when someone names it as dance.

In sum, by being and representing a logic of bodily becoming, dancing appears as religion, as expressing a *unity of life*. An individ- ual exercises and acquires power for himself by making move- ments—kinetic images—that express an infinite web of self and humanity within which his dancing is suspended. In this way, in so far as dancing engages as its medium the medium through which humans live, whenever a person dances, his action affords some glimpse of the potency of dancing to project an image of life as a "unity"—that is, to conduct an experience of order and of power in its paradoxical form. To this extent, dancing, van der Leeuw avers, is "religious in itself [*van zelf religieus*], even when specifically reli- gious objectives are lacking" (S 12; W 10).

Nevertheless, this account of dancing as bodily movement is only part of van der Leeuw's story. As noted, a dancer never appears as an abstract individual. She is always exercising her physical conscious- ness in a concrete time and place, through particular webs of cultural meaning. Further explanation of how the logic of bodily becoming works requires attention to this second dimension of dance—culture.

DANCE AS CULTURE

Van der Leeuw's account of dance as able to allow otherwise disparate moments of bodily life to appear in relation to one another is devel- oped further in his discussion of dance as culture.[5] Van der Leeuw maps a circular relationship between dance and culture: he introduces his concept of culture using images of dance in order to set forth a framework for examining dance as a manifestation of culture. In this analysis, dance appears as one instance of culture by enabling an appearance of culture in the form of a unity—process and product in the same moment. In this way, dance performs a cultural, not just a bodily reflexivity. Dance demonstrates its phenomenological connection with religion by displaying the rhythms that van der Leeuw perceives as constituting culture—what I call a spiral of discovery and response.

What then is culture and how does dancing appear to enact its unity? Van der Leeuw uses the Dutch *beschaving*, with the sense of "grinding to a finish," to represent the action humans take in creating and making real the selves and the worlds in which they live.[6] Culture is "the domain of what is properly human, of the man who does not simply accept the world as he finds it, but rather transforms it into his own world" (S 13; W 32). While van der Leeuw's concept of culture includes the idea of a "symbolic universe" within which human meaning is possible, it refers most generally to the *action* of participating in the generation of such universes, and only secondly, the material, intellectual, and emotional fruits of that laboring.[7] Culture is a *process* that finds expression in the making of cultural forms be they ideas, institutions, language, symbols, or technology.[8]

In describing this process, van der Leeuw draws on images of dance. He writes:

> Culture is the movement of man through nature. In the process, three main possibilities are realized: man overcomes the world and masters it, succeeding with the help of his magic and his science, which are related to each other and coincide to a degree with each other; or he controls his dependence on the powers of this world, either by subjecting himself to them [and] allowing himself to be ruled, doing this in a state of enthusiasm or ecstasy; or he seeks for himself a place outside the course of the world which allows him to observe, and this he does in art, in science, and in contemplation . . . Man tries to

stride, heavily and emphatically, to hover, light and high, or to
move along calmly, and more or less conscious of responsibility.
(S 14; W 12-13)

As the "movement of man," culture represents the actions through
which a person relates to his natural and social environments, and
works out a sense of self in relation to a sense of world.⁹ This movement, moreover, appears to van der Leeuw in the form of particular
possibilities or "styles." These styles are intellectual and emotional,
and van der Leeuw's use of movement metaphors signals sensory and
kinesthetic dimensions as well. As the following analyses of these
styles suggests, for van der Leeuw, culture resembles an open-ended
dialectical interplay between forms of reason and experience.

Before undertaking this analysis, however, it is important to note
that van der Leeuw couples his account of culture as a form of dance
with an enhanced definition of dance as a form of culture. Dance is a
singular manifestation "within the totality of culture" (S 14; W 13).
Note the parallels:

> The dance is indeed the movement [*gang*] of man in the literal
> sense, but it is not his natural movement [*zooals hij reilt en
> zeilt*— lock, stock and barrel], being rather the specifically
> human movement created by him. It is ordered movement
> [*geordende gang*]. The dance is a movement of the self in a pur-
> poseful, definite manner. It is walking the way we walked as
> children, with one foot on the sidewalk and the other in the
> street; or three steps forward on the right foot then one on the
> left. In the dance, man discovers the rhythm of the motion
> [*beweging*] that surrounds him, just as it surrounds another
> man or an animal or a star. He discovers the rhythm and invents
> a response, but it is a response that has its own forms, that is
> stylized and ordered. He does with motion [*beweging*] the same
> thing that he does with a shape when he carves or chisels, draws
> or paints. He places his own movements [*beweging*] and those

of the creatures which surround him into an ordered whole. (S 14; W 13)

By emphasizing that dance is not "lock, stock and barrel" movement, van der Leeuw locates dance as a creative act against those who might dismiss it as natural or animal, and thus, accidental to the work of culture.[10] The movement that appears as dance is *beautiful*—it appears as "stylized and ordered." As ordered, it embodies human intention and expresses human need; it refers to movements that humans perform with consciousness (even if spontaneously), in shapes that may be recognized within a culture as dance (even when improvised).

Yet, for van der Leeuw, the value of dance as a moment in culture does not lie in particular steps but rather in the way in which dancing discloses the phenomenological structure that characterizes culture itself. Dance enacts a spiraling process of discovery and response, a response that "has its own forms." For van der Leeuw, dance makes visible the process in which humans recreate the forms of their experience in ways that make real a world.

In the quotation above, van der Leeuw tells this story. A human being is one who, from her earliest moments of awareness, senses rhythms in her self/world (undifferentiated at first). She is born into the styles and movement patterns characteristic of a given culture and its geography. As she matures, she discovers rhythms as her sensitivity to those akin to the ones with which she is familiar increases. These rhythms educate her senses. Exploring these movements through the movements of her own body, she "invents a response." She dances. Her dances thus represent her recreation of (her relationship to) the rhythms she senses. They also represent the attention and effort she must engage in order to craft her response. In this way, her movement responses enact—and realize—a sense of her self as a function of her relation to her community and larger world. She grows into an adult member of her community by participating in the ongoing evolution (or revolution) of its cultural styles.

With this definition of dance as culture, van der Leeuw maps the interdependence of the logic of bodily becoming (described above) and the spiral of discovery and response. The former enables the latter; the latter informs the former. As a person discovers rhythms and invents a kinetic response, he moves. He develops strength, facility, and physical consciousness, and invests these resources in further acts of discovery and kinetic image making. In dance, then, a person not only expresses a unity of bodily life, and (as we shall see) a unity of cultural life, he also enacts their interdependence. In dance, a person appears as the process of becoming himself in and through the process of creating culture. For this reason, van der Leeuw concludes, regardless of content or theme or context or steps, the act of dancing both is and makes visible a unity of life—the constitutive, evolving coordination of self and world that culture is. In such instances what appears as dance appears as religion. Where bodily becoming continues, the culture-spiral never ends.

The following discussion of the three styles in which dance as culture appears to van der Leeuw traces this interdependence of body and culture. While van der Leeuw notes that the three styles of culture he names may be present in every hour and every moment of life, he nevertheless finds the distinctions among them helpful for organizing a variety of dances catalogued in historical records (S 14; W 13). Each style represents a different form in which a dancer enacts the culture-spiral of discovery and response, and thus highlights a different structural relation linking appearances of "dance" and "religion." A discussion of each generates further conceptual resources for scholars interested in theorizing religion and dance.

Striding

To begin, striding marks a style of dancing that appears as an effort to establish mastery over "the world" through a process of *imitating* the movements of some perceived force or power, whether animal, human, natural, or supernatural. These dances may involve masks and pantomime and often occur in the shape of a ring.

In an effort to understand why humans dance in imitation of a wolf, an ancestor, or the Hindu god Siva, van der Leeuw explores the idea that a dancer who does so seeks to secure for herself the power of an entity she perceives as other by mastering the rhythms that appear to her as characterizing that other. He writes:

> The rhythm must be discovered; then the dance arises, which imposes it on the environment, thereby drawing the environment into the movement as well. This is what is meant when the dance is spoken of as a "motion-magic." This is not a beautiful word, but it makes the situation clear. Man perceives the motion of the surrounding environment and then, in his turn, forces it upon the world after his own fashion. (S 15; W 14)

What is imitated in these dances is not the animal or god "itself," but the form of the rhythm as ascertained and recreated by a dancer. By making an image of the form in which an animal (for example) appears to her, she in effect reproduces her relation to the animal. Or rather, she enacts that relationship—she offers a picture of her relation to that animal which becomes true through her dancing as the condition for that dancing. It is in this sense that van der Leeuw describes such dancing as "forcing" a rhythmic image upon the world: the dance represents the meaning of the animal in terms of its relation to the dancer. The dance is *"een daad van verovering*—'a deed of conquering.'"[11]

The effect of such image making, as van der Leeuw contends, is that a dancer is able to appropriate the power of the force whose appearance to him he recreates in the dance as his own. He does so by making its movements—that is, representing his relationship to it as one characterized by mastery. As van der Leeuw avers: "Everywhere in the world, men assume the nature of animals, the dead, or the gods, in order to make sure, by means of the dance, that whatever is desired of them will be performed" (S 18; W 39). In this analysis, van der Leeuw does not judge whether a dancer actually changes the action of a god. As a phenomenologist, he seeks to understand what it means for dancing to appear to someone as having this potency. As he explains, in so far as a dancer masters the god's movement by making visible this image of their relationship, then whatever a god does may be interpreted in terms of "whatever is desired." Even if a god seems to act against what is desired, the meaning of those events may be interpreted in terms of that god's power.[12]

This striding style, van der Leeuw insists, is not limited to animal and masked dances. In so-called modern societies, erotic couple or pair dances [*paardans*] provide another excellent example. From this perspective, where a couple dance such as the waltz or fox trot imitates the movements of lovemaking, the dancers enact the relational context within which either one of the partner's future actions—whether argumentative or affectionate—will have meaning for the other. Their dancing imitates and appropriates the power of love as defining the reality of their relationship.

So then, how does the act of mastering the rhythms of an other's appearance effect a transfer of power from that animal, god, or tradition to the person dancing? Van der Leeuw describes at least two rhythms or paradoxes that govern this style spiral of discovery and response: the rhythms of mastery and submission, and proximity and distance. First, the process of discovery prerequisite to inventing and performing an imitative or striding dance entails a period of submission to the observed force. The form must be mastered. A person watches and learns and finds in her own sensibility the capacity to make movements that mirror those she observes in the animal, god, or tradition. The paradox is this: the degree of mastery which a person is able to command appears in proportion to the care with which she attends to the forms of the other whose power she intends to appropriate. In turn, given the logic of bodily becoming described above, as a dancer finds the shapes of will and intent that enable her to make the rhythmic movements that appear to her, she expresses her own power. Her own agency appears as enabled by the act of learning to make the movements of the other. "By dancing the movements of the animals," van der Leeuw writes, a human "becomes master of the animal rhythm. He subjects to himself the order of the animals, he adds the power of the animals [*de macht der dieren schakelt*] to his own."[13] The discipline required to add the power of an animal to her own is subjection—in its double sense. The act of mastering the forms transforms the dancer into someone capable of making the desired movements. She enacts her/its power.

This rhythm of submission and mastery implies a second and related paradox that facilitates the transfer of power from animal, natural, or supernatural force to dancer in striding dances: proximity and distance. A successful period of tutelage depends on a dancer's *desire* for relationship with what he dances. The dancer's desire motivates his act of submission and *also* influences what he does and does not notice in the process of studying. As he becomes more invested in what appears to him, drawing more of his kinetic experience into his response, his representations of a god's movements reflect more of the other *and* more of his own receptive, kinetic ability. As van der Leeuw confirms, the image making involved in art is not the same as making a *copy*: "Art is not an imitation [*nabootsing*] of the movement of life. Art has its own movement" (S 86; W 116). Where desire is at work, imitation is impossible. In dancing, a dancer creates a new movement—one that expresses his desire for relation to that with which he dances. Yet this desire to draw as closely as possible to the object, to approximate its movements exactly, produces the distinctive virtuosity of an individual dancer. As he loses his sense of subjectivity to the rhythms he seeks to master, he expresses more strongly and more precisely his self in relation to the god as master of its movements. Even where the identity of the individual is hidden beneath a mask, his ability to make the movements empowers his particular embodiment as a conduit for the force that mask represents. His mimetic dancing serves, in other words, to make the other *other*. This intimate distance between dancer and danced, image and imaged, only intensifies as the spiral of tutelage and mastery continues.

By enacting these rhythms of submission and mastery, proximity and distance, mimetic dances effect and represent the process by which humans realize an image of order—a sense of self in relation to world—that they desire. Regardless of how wild or indifferent to human living her dancing depicts a given force as being, when a person submits herself to it and dances it, she demonstrates her mastery over the form of its appearance.

Van der Leeuw surmises why it makes sense, given the way in which striding dances enact the unity of cultural life, that these dances appear to him as religion. Dancing appears as religion by laying claim not only to the horizon within which the real appears, but also to the power of horizon making. He summarizes:

> The religious character of the dance is shown most clearly in the dance pantomime . . . Through imitation [*nabootsing*], the power of the original act is transferred to a new act. For the primitive mind, the representation of the action is realistically bound up with what is represented. The war dance, accordingly, is a kind of war, and its movement influences the outcome . . . But the case is no different with the religious in the narrow sense than it is with these—again, in our eyes—secular things . . . The great movement of death and life is imitated and made dependable in the dance [*De groote gang van dood en leven wordt in den dans nageboost en verzekerd*]. (S 17-8; 38)

Dancing makes this great movement of life and death "dependable" by recreating the form in which it appears to a dancer in a way which enables her or those who watch her to experience life's movements as "dependable," as comprising an "order." By dancing, a person imposes this order onto life, concealing the reality her dance purports to reveal. At the same time, however, the person is dancing, she is becoming her bodily self by inventing her response to the rhythms of life and drawing upon their power to fund and articulate her own.

According to van der Leeuw, it is by way of this process that dancing rehearses a human's ability to respond to whatever uncanny powers interrupt his own projects and goals. He writes: "After the dance comes the sowing and plowing, and not rarely, mating. But the dance itself stands alone. It is game, art, ritual. It contains [*dwingt*—'compels or constrains'] reality, but it is not reality . . . Man interpolates, so to speak, the path of the stars into his own path" (S 22; W 19-20). The dance is "not [the] reality" of what it represents: a planting dance cannot substitute for the act of putting seeds in the ground. Yet, as process and product of culture, dancing "compels and constrains" even the "path of the stars" by exercising the human capacity for imitating reality, for making (its) meaning. Dance "stands alone" as "its own articulation" alongside other forms of culture as the activity that reveals the rhythm of discovery and response within which all human action, thought, and meaning arise. The kinetic images of a dance are increments of power.

Hovering, Light and High

The second style that van der Leeuw describes in his account of dance as expressing the unity of cultural life is to "hover, light and high" (S14; W 12-13). Under this name, van der Leeuw attends to the transformations wrought in the sensory space of a body by the physical action of making dance movements. He explains that

> it is not only mask and pantomime which bring the *other* nearer, but also the movement itself . . . there is another kind of freeing, which we can understand today, that which comes through frenzy or ecstasy. With this, we have come to the second kind of movement, that of hovering. In the ecstatic dance, too, one dances for

the good things of life. The two sorts cannot be separated; only the rhythm is different. We are no longer concerned with the round dance and its well-defined center, but with the whirl of the leaves. Here, man does not subjugate the world by mastering a rhythm, but by being himself caught up in and ruled by this rhythm. (S 24; W 41, 22-3)

Where the efficacy of mimetic dances derives from the effort required to master an image of an other's rhythm, the efficacy of hovering movement derives from the experience of surrendering to the whirl of movement itself. Driving rhythms beat and breathe the dancer into a place where she experiences herself grasped by power greater than herself—the power represented in and by the rhythms she dances. Repetitive movements serve to dissolve her awareness of the sensible boundaries distinguishing self from the dance, soul from body from surroundings. As van der Leeuw writes, "the dance is a compulsion which assumes control of the man, a madness sweeping him along. The dancer does not move actively, but floats or hovers passively . . . The man 'is danced'" (S 25; W 23). The ecstatic dancer, in effect, loses her self to the dance; the dance becomes the dancer.

As a dancer "is danced," however, he is not simply negated but, following the logic of bodily becoming, he is transformed. What is reborn through the dancing itself is not strictly speaking a "self," but rather a heightened sensory awareness of total immersion in a vibrating web of life—a sense of hovering, of being buoyed by currents of living energy. Van der Leeuw describes this sense as one of being suspended or being held in suspense, light and high (S 14; W 12-13). As a dancer dances, he exercises and cultivates a vulnerability to being moved by some power other than himself. Describing the dancing of the Kwakiutl Indians, van der Leeuw writes:

The compulsive transition to the other, to the nonhuman, is very apparent here. The sharp rhythm, the monotonous movement, the furious tempo, all put the dancer beside [or "outside"] himself. And at all times, man has believed that the negation of self has brought him closer to a higher life. Whoever has lost his self has room for God. (S 26; W 41)

In the style of hovering, then, dance appears to enact a unity of culture in so far as the dancing effects an experience in which all life and all forms and expressions and manifestations of culture are swept away. In this way, ecstatic dance makes apparent the common transitory ephemeral character and inevitable end of all representations of self and world. Ecstatic dance brings dancers to the brink of that moment described in Chapter 6 as becoming understood, where a new round of creation can begin. For historical examples of such "ecstatic dance" [*de extatische dans*], van der Leeuw refers to dances practiced by the Sufi dervishes, as well as followers of the Greek Dionysus and the Hindu god Siva. He also cites the Franciscan ecstatic, Jacopone da Todi, whose *Laude* includes the line: "Everyone who loves the Lord, come to the dance and sing of love. May he come to the dance, completely caught up by love" (S 26; W 25).

A question arises: is van der Leeuw contradicting himself? The two culture "paths" between religion and dance he identifies seem to move in opposite directions: striding or mimetic dances impose rhythmic order onto the self-world relation; hovering dances dissolve the sensible boundaries that orient humans within "reality." Van der Leeuw insists that pantomime reveals the "religious character" of dance most clearly, and then contends that all dance is "ecstatic" (S 25; W 23). Which is it?

A clue lies in the spiral of discovery and response characteristic of culture that each style animates, though differently. As van der Leeuw explains:

To understand the psychology of the dance and to see at the same time its connection with religion, we must look upon its rhythm as motion and response, the seizing of life and the discarding of life [*het leven grijpend en het leven wegwerpend*].

> The rhythm unfolds in a double manner. By constraining life,
> seizing it and limiting it, rhythm gives strength [*macht*] to life
> ... rhythm moves the feet, the spirit, and the gods. It is the
> pulse of animal life, the heartbeat of our spiritual life, the
> movement [*beweging*] of the world and the course of the gods.
> (S 27; W 42)

All dances—circular or whirling, mimetic or ecstatic—participate in
the same double rhythm of motion and response, affirmation and
ecstasy, seizing and discarding. Dancing seizes or grasps "life" by
imposing and making real an order binding dancer to world; dancing
discards or lets go of "life" as a dancer repeatedly loses herself and her
sense of form. The seizing and the discarding happen in every dance,
in every moment of dancing, and define the process though which a
dance occurs in time. Even in whirling dances, it is the seizing of life
into the form of a rhythm that catalyzes an experience of boundary
dissolution; even in the mimetic dances, it is the loss of the form of
the self to the form of the other in the moment of subjection that
secures the transfer of power from other to self. The difference
between the two styles, then, is one of direction: striding moves
towards form; whirling moves towards formlessness, each engaging
the tension between seizing and discarding in order to move. By
being and representing the interdependent, spiraling creation and dissolution of forms constitutive of all cultural forms, ecstatic and
mimetic dances appear as religion.

Walking, More or Less Responsibly

In fleshing out his phenomenological account of dance as expressing
culture, van der Leeuw designates a third style of movement: walking
contemplatively, or stepping aside and pondering, "more or less
responsibly" (S 14; W 12-13). Initially, this movement style does not
seem to designate "dance" at all. Any striding is reigned in and hov-

ering has settled to earth, tethered into the movements of a walk. Moreover, the value of this walking seems to lie in its ability to nourish mental movements of contemplation. It describes a movement of stopping the dance, stepping outside its sphere of action, and contemplating. Many of the historical examples van der Leeuw includes as moments under this structure are drawn from Christian history or its Gnostic representatives. He cites the Christian Fathers and medieval saints for whom the "whole of Christian life is thought of as a dance" (S 30; W 28). He identifies mystics who contemplate dance in pursuit of religious insight, and theologians who invoke dance to describe salvation. In these cases, more often than not, persons call upon an image of dance to buttress a distinction between a heavenly realm where humans dance with angels, and an earthly realm in which humans do not and cannot dance.

Yet, in introducing this third style of movement as dance, van der Leeuw teases out a formal element of dancing which is as necessary to its performance as the movements of seizing and discarding life: stillness. As evident already, every form of every dance represents a constraint of available movement possibilities—a style. The movement of dance is ordered. Any given style is selected from among an infinite array of movement possibilities; it appears as a form belonging to this person and culture and not another, and when rehearsed over the course of a lifetime, it develops the bodies who practice it into bodies capable of performing it.[14] Implicit, then, within the phenomenological form of a dance style is the possibility that the ordering so constrains the movement that a dancer stops and freezes into a fixed image of himself. For the dance to continue, of course, he must discard that image, seize another, and empty himself into its unfolding in space and time. Van der Leeuw's genius is to see this still point in dance movement—where dance appears as an image of itself—as necessarily given in the double rhythm of dance itself. Contemplating dance images thus appears to him as a *style* of *dancing*.

The fruits of this naming are several, and exploring them will draw together the preceding discussions of dance as a logic of bodily becoming and dance as striding and hovering culture. In brief, van der Leeuw provides himself with the means for: first, interpreting images of dance in visual art, literature, and music as evidence for the internal connections he seeks between dance and religion; second, identifying structural relations linking dance to the other arts; and third, justifying his project of writing about dance and religion for his chosen audience—members of the Dutch Reformed Church, in particular, and citizens of modern societies in general—with the intent of priming their desire to appreciate dance as "religion."

Interpreting dance imagery. In approaching the contemplation of dance images as a third style of dancing, van der Leeuw is able to mobilize his phenomenological analyses of dance *practice* (i.e., striding and hovering) as keys to interpreting the visual and verbal images of dance shared by members of a religious tradition that does not endorse actual dancing. A prominent example is van der Leeuw's reading of the second-century Gnostic text, "The Acts of John." In this account of the night before Jesus' crucifixion, Jesus stands in the center of a circle of disciples. They revolve around him. He calls; they respond. He says to them: "Whoever does not dance will not know what will happen."[15] As van der Leeuw interprets,

> The dance becomes contemplative and reflects the highest form of movement, the movement of God. The most eloquent example of such a dance of mystic contemplation is the image of the dancing Christ, which was current in Gnostic circles during the early centuries of our era. The movement of God's love in Christ [*De beweging der liefde Gods in Christus*] is apprehended as a dance which Christ performs with his twelve disciples. (S 29; W 27)

Whether or not Jesus actually danced with his disciples (instead of celebrating the Last Supper as canonical gospels report) funds scholarly debates.[16] For van der Leeuw, answering the question is the responsibility of a historian, not a phenomenologist. What is undeniable is that the text depicts an *image* of Christ dancing with his disciples, and van der Leeuw asks about its meaning in the text itself. To van der Leeuw's eyes, the dance appears as a ring dance, a mimetic dance, whose meaning—as an image—can be understood by reading the relationship between the dancing Christ and his dancing disciples through the paradoxical rhythms of submission and mastery, proximity and distance. In so far as the disciples *discover* Christ dancing, their desire is stirred to imitate the form in which Christ appears to them, as the "movement of God's love" in him for them. They *respond* by finding within themselves the capacity to entertain similar movements for others. Christ's words quoted above support this interpretation: in seeking to move like Christ, they will move toward Christ, and come to know the love of God moving toward them and in them. As they recreate in themselves the forms in which Christ appears to them, then, humans "know what will happen"; they will know that their relationship to God is consummated in mutual love.

In this interpretation, van der Leeuw illuminates the dance imagery as integral to the meaning of the text: in so far as the text represents dancing as essential to knowing, so the disciples' action in awakening their own movement capacity—their capacity to love—is essential to the process of imitating Christ. Those who call themselves disciples must submit themselves to the rhythmic forms in which Christ appears to them in order to learn to exercise their own agency; they express themselves as they master the movements of love Christ demonstrates. Dancing thus appears as a metaphor describing the process of coming to know God—a metaphor whose efficacy presumes an experience of dancing embedded in cultural and bodily memory. Actually doing a dance remains a meaningful idea.

By mobilizing his phenomenological understanding of mimetic or striding dances in this example, van der Leeuw is able to interpret the dance imagery of the text as evidence of a structural connection between dance and religion regardless of whether dancing ever actually occurred. In this instance, the author's choice of dance as the paradigm for representing a human relation to God relies upon and expresses a perception of dancing as enacting a unity of (bodily and cultural) life. Van der Leeuw's interpretation of the text may also suggest why it proved threatening to Christian teachers interested in consolidating the authority of the church: the link between knowing God and dancing lies in the idea of participation. Dancing signals a knowing in which a person must exercise his individual embodiment—his desire, will, and experience—over and against institutional authority, as the medium for receiving an experience of otherly power or Love moving in him.

Relating the arts. The contemplation of dance as an image, when itself considered as a structural possibility given in dancing itself, holds a second benefit: it enables van der Leeuw to disclose the structural associations through which the various arts appear in relation to one another as "art." Where dance includes the movement of stilling movement into an image, then dance includes an oscillating rhythm between image and movement common to all art, and all forms of communication in general. Dance appears as the source, and *telos,* the enabling matrix of other arts.

First, structurally speaking, where dance enacts culture—a spiral of discovery and response, the creation and dissolution of form— dance is and represents the source of every act that appears as an impression or expression of beauty. As van der Leeuw writes, "every art is movement" (S 155; W 205) and, "movement is in all art, essential."[17] In practicing an art, artists further constrain or stylize the encultured, bodily movement which dancing is, in order to isolate one of the sensory elements produced by that movement as their medium. An artist practices bodily movements that develop the expressive capacity of one or several of these elements. The rhythms and sounds articulated in words and music, the images, shapes, and colors arrested in visual art and sculpture, or the expansion through space fixed by architecture all appear as constitutive elements of the most basic dance movement. For this reason, van der Leeuw will say, dance as *beschaving* "enables, in turn, other arts to come into being: music, song, drama" (S 12; W 11).

At the same time, the relationship between dance and other arts is *structural*, not chronological, logical, or historical; it must be read as moving in two directions.[18] Dance is revealed as enabling matrix only when arrested in the form of an image and juxtaposed alongside the other arts it always already engenders. In other words, the image of dance as matrix emerges coextensive with the arts it purportedly enables.

Further, not only does dance appear as the matrix of the arts, but by appearing as both movement and image, dancing reveals the structural or constitutive principle that marks art as art—what van der Leeuw calls a "paradox of expression" (S 141; W 188). This paradox is a version of the paradox of revelation and concealment, focused on the act of expressing. In a nutshell: images fix movement; movement dissolves images, and any act of expression or communication regardless of the medium requires some combination of both. Without the image, movement has no form; without movement, an image has no life. In short, as van der Leeuw explains, an image is another name for a phenomenon: a human recreation of the form in which something *appears* to someone. What is concealed in the image is the movement, the life, that the image is intended to reveal. For this reason, van der Leeuw can say both that movement is "essential in all the arts" (S 253; W 419-20), and that the image is the "principle of art in its totality" (S 192; W 339).

Van der Leeuw provides his most complete account of the paradox of expression in his discussion on the visual arts. Here he offers a description of an image that pertains to those found in dance and of dance:

> An image is something which can be seen and touched; it has firm contours and a particular nature. It is neither thought nor "idea" but harsh [*harde* or hard] reality. But it is also not simply a thing, an object. It takes its nature from the fact that it tries to express, reproduce something. . . . its reality coincides with another reality. . . . "It resembles". . . . The relationship between both realities is neither accidentally nor purposely caused. The picture is not something arbitrary, but the essence of what is represented, its manifestation, its form of appearance. (S 306; W 307-8)

The "reality" which an image represents is already "a visionary form [*een geziene gestalte*—a form which is seen]," that is, an appearance to someone of something (S 156; W 208). In this sense, an image is always already an image of an image, recreated through a conscious attempt to re-experience the form of the initial appearance. Thus, an image is an "expression of a remarkable double experience"— a third thing, not the object and not a subject's fiction, but an effort to reproduce the appearance of the former for the latter. Van der Leeuw elaborates: "Things do not exist, at least man has no approach, if they are not represented. Only what is represented as an image in a second reality has existence. . . . There is no reality besides that which is consummated in an image" (S 305; W 306). Image making allows for an approach, even as it conceals any originary experience. The "essence" of an image is its manifestation, the form of its appearance.

Yet, over and again in his discussion of images, van der Leeuw issues a warning. In so far as an image wrenches visibility from a never-ending stream of life—the chaotic maze of the given—then "representation always moves between two dangers: the perfection of the image (the autonomy of what is depicted) and the disappearance of the image" (S 187; W 252). When a person holds an image too lightly, not giving it any weight to compel or constrain reality, then the image retains too close a connection to movement; the image may be overwhelmed by the "undertow" of dance, whose rhythm and movement succeed in "banishing visibility" (S 291; W 282). Conversely, when a person holds an image too tightly, embracing it as reality, she denies its participation in the paradox of revelation and concealment. She denies its source in movement and thus its role in enabling intelligibility. Van der Leeuw contends, the "freezing of motion . . . can change at any moment . . . to the denial of movement" with the effect that the movement of life "takes on an absolute character and does not leave room for any other possibilities. It binds the free imagination [*de vrije verbeelding*]" (S 178; W 240).

In sum, any image—whether kinetic, visual, or logical—enables communication only in so far as the person using it or receiving it is able to appreciate the image as an image of an image—a recreation of an appearance to someone of some moment in the stream of life: "What does not appear before our eyes as an image we do not perceive within this world as powerful" (S 306; W 308). Yet, a perfect image is an idol. It occludes the rhythms of understanding—the fluid exchange between subject and object, the interplay of self and world within which meanings appear and images arise; as van der Leeuw says, "in the perfect image, there is nothing more to see" (S 187; W 253). The aim, in terms discussed in Part 1, is to allow a dialectical interplay—a mutually generating movement—between the image-making power of reason and the ever-active flux of experience.

In so far as dancing enacts this tension between image and movement making, what the arts share—their one-ness—is a relation to dancing that is at once a relation to religion. Each art earns its potency for conducting experiences of obtruding, dislocating power through the element of dance which that art stylizes as its distinguishing feature. Conversely, the potential for each aesthetic product to appear as religion depends upon the abilities of its makers, performers, and appreciators to *remember* the structural relations linking the appearance of the aesthetic object to beautiful movement. In other words, each art must remember its structural link with dance in order to guard against the two dangers of expression—fixing or dissolving images.

Take drama, for example. Drama emerges, for van der Leeuw, when "movement meets countermovement" (S 78; W 105). The opposition generates tension between characters; the creative figuring of this tension makes drama "drama." Based on this formal link, van der Leeuw claims that dance "is beyond doubt the art which plays the most important role in the structure of the drama. The drama can do without words and without music, but never without movement" (S 78; W 105). Drama, like dance, is, illuminates, and advances the capacity for enacting the great rhythms of life and death: "Life and death as they occur in nature and in the life of mankind, the eternal cycle [*omslag*—'ceremony, fuss'] of life to death, death to life, the monotonous but heart-stirring rhythm which pulses everywhere, within us and around us, are represented *dramatically* as movement and countermovement."[19]

Through this analysis of drama as a structural derivative of dancing, van der Leeuw concludes that the religious potency of drama is lost unless the actor remembers those elements of his image-making that bind him to the dancer: an actor engages his medium of life in surrendering to the rhythmic forms that appear to him (in the shape of a character or role), recreating his perception of those forms, mastering them, drawing their life force into his own, and expressing himself through them. An actor must become himself by playing not the "role of a man, but the role of a role" (S 89; W 121). Only then, van der Leeuw avers, "can one speak of high art and of a broadening and deepening which lead to the boundary of earthly existence" (S 106; W 144).

In *Sacred and Profane Beauty,* van der Leeuw performs similar analyses with each art. At each turn, he isolates the element of dance in that art that marks both its derivation and distance from dance, and thus its internal relation to religion. Briefly, architecture, in its construction of living spaces, develops the "principle of creation [*het element der schepping*]" evident in the way dance movement defines the self-world relation (S 209; W 359). Music mobilizes the interplay of silence and sound, best evoking what van der Leeuw calls the "paradox of expression," or the "great struggle" of reaching for an inexpressible other.[20] Words, in turn, as they engage and direct the experiences of the writer, represent the service [*Dienst*]—the paradox of submission and mastery—which inspiration demands (S 148-9; W 198-9). Finally, the visual image, as noted, represents "the principle of art in its totality" as a process of arresting movement into images (S 192; W 339). In each case, to the extent that a given art sustains (while elaborating) whatever structural links it bears to dance, the art appears in its distinctive manner as art and demonstrates an ability to occasion paradoxical expressions of power.

Through the analysis of dance as an image of movement, then, van der Leeuw makes his case for the importance of dancing: the health of the arts as impressions and expressions of beauty in any given society depends upon the ability of the society's members to conceive of dance as one art, alongside other arts. In and through dance, people can comprehend the common participation of the arts in the spiraling movements of bodily and cultural life. If they do not attend to dance as art, members of a given society will not be confronted with an experience in which the arts coincide. In so far as people are not educated through dance to conceive the structural relations linking the arts to one another, then they will also miss the potential of each art to appear as religion. The refusal to embrace dance as art enables and perpetuates one-sided conceptions of art and religion as representing discrete and potentially opposing spheres of life. Consciousness of dance as religion requires the double movement of dance itself: people must step outside of the dance and contemplate its structural connectedness with the other arts, while acknowledging that their ability to step aside and contemplate the dance as object is itself given in the phenomenal form of dance itself.

206 Between Dancing and Writing

Justifying writing. By interpreting dance imagery as evidence of the structural connections between art and religion, and by disclosing the unity of the arts via the paradox of expression, van der Leeuw secures a third and related fruit from naming his third style of dance: justification for (his own) thinking and writing about dancing—that is, for making verbal images of dance. A dance image, while signaling the death of dance, is also a fossil, a memory of a living form. In so far as any text or art-bound image of dance implicitly acknowledges the religious potency of dance practice, then the appearance of that image in writing defines a trajectory from dance to image that can and must be reversed. For van der Leeuw, the responsibility for writing about dance as an expression of life falls onto the shoulders of contemporary scholars of religion.

What distinguishes a dance image that rekindles a desire to dance from dance imagery that arrests actual dancing? The difference lies in the attitude or consciousness of the person to whom it appears. For van der Leeuw, a phenomenologist who understands dancing as enacting a rhythmic spiral of discovery and response through the becoming of individual bodies can grasp how any one image of dance, stilled and contemplated, has meaning (at least in part) by virtue of how it participates in this rhythmic spiral. As van der Leeuw notes: "The image is not immobile; rather it is petrified movement [*gestremde beweging*]."[21] By perceiving an image as petrified move-ment, a scholar remembers the rhythmic context—the living reality—that enables the image to have meaning as "dance." She remembers that, powerful as they are, words and images cannot substitute for the transformation of a person's experiential capacity that occurs in and through the practice of mimetic and ecstatic dances. Her words and images about dance call attention to dance as *its own* articulation, as a medium of experience and expression. To see an image of dance as petrified movement, then, is to acknowledge an irreducible structural tension between writing and dancing. Dancing exercises and projects a unity (image and movement) of what the practice of writing holds apart (image and movement).

A scholar with this consciousness who seeks to write about dance will develop a self-consciousness of his writing as an embodied practice. Recounting his own experience, van der Leeuw explains:

> In writing about the dance, I discovered that, even more than in the other arts, participation is necessary if it is to be understood. With the spoken or written word, little can be explained when the point is to appreciate the rhythm and imitate it. And yet the word is able to follow the dance, at a distance; for the word itself is only one of the many forms of human expression (like music) which, though they have their independent life and rules, cannot be separated from the dance, and in comparison to it are less broad, less comprehensive, less totalitarian (S 12; W 11).

It is the experience of writing that leads van der Leeuw to the conclusion that understanding dance requires *participation*—learning, practicing, and performing the rhythms of a given style. The practice of writing, in other words, does not guarantee its own success when the object is dance. However, van der Leeuw is also aware that his ability even to notice this difference between dancing and writing witnesses to what dancing and writing share: participation in the paradox of expression common to all forms of human communication. The implication, then, is that the experience of writing about dance awakens van der Leeuw to the situation Johannes de Silentio describes: the ways in which the practice of writing as itself rhythmic bodily movement both—and at the same time—enables and forecloses avenues of understanding religion and dance.

One implication of this phenomenological relationship between dancing and writing that van der Leeuw discovers is that writing about dance may be essential for understanding religion in its phenomenal forms and as a concept. For one, when confronted with the phenomenon of dance, scholars are constantly reminded not to make the theological error of claiming that whatever they can write about religion or a religious phenomenon can ever be a "last word." In other words, by writing about dancing, scholars can come to appreciate their own writing activity as a species of dancing—one that has developed the imaging dimension of dance, sacrificing "totalitarian" breadth for precision.

Further, in writing about dance as religion, scholars can also call attention to the phenomenological relationship between dance and religion that the forms of modern culture, as Chapter 9 explains, both presuppose and deny. They become aware of how their theories of religion perpetuate a distinction between writing and dancing; they become aware of how much of what passes in the world as dancing cannot *appear* to them. In making such arguments, van der Leeuw is not offering a theological defense of dance with reference to a sacred "Unity." He is offering a nuanced analysis of how scholars who rely on the practice of writing to secure a distance from theology inevitably devalue dance in relation to what appears through their practice as "religion."

Even so, van der Leeuw is cautious in his recommendations. The point of writing about dance in relation to religion is not to orchestrate a return to a time in which people danced religion. From a phenomenological perspective, complete return is structurally impossible (S 70; W 94). Van der Leeuw confirms that "we have lost the dance as an element of culture almost completely . . . Dance as an art form, as pure entertainment, is a fossil of the living dance, which once had its own, much more inclusive social function [*levensfunctie*]" (S 32-3; W 31). He goes on: "In a word, we have lost the unity of life [*levenseenheid*]" (S 33; W 35). That is, we have lost the ability to perceive dance as enacting the unity of life. In so doing, we have lost the ability to appreciate the structural relations binding dance to the arts and the arts to one another. We have lost consciousness of writing itself as a species of dancing. To this extent we convince ourselves that writing can and should arrest the movement of theology. In response, van der Leeuw urges us to write about dance as religion in order to rehabilitate dance in the consciousness of readers and thereby open up the possibility for creating new forms of dance and religion responsive to the concerns of our time. Through writing about dance, he suggests, we can begin to think about writing and dancing as engaged in an irreducible, dialectical interplay—an ongoing exchange of *petrified movement* and *kinetic images*—enabling religious studies.

In *Sacred and Profane Beauty,* van der Leeuw practices what he counsels others to do. He writes about dance. He deploys his phenomenological account of dance as expressing a unity of life in order to perceive and understand other historical moments in which dance and religion appear in relation to one another. He finds at least four other phenomenological structures characterizing these moments. These remaining four occupy Chapter 9.

Marking Boundaries
Dance against Religion

When van der Leeuw turns to elaborate four other phenomenological nets he has woven in his efforts to write about relationships between dance and religion appearing in human history, the significance of the first net—namely the unity of dance and religion—emerges with greater clarity. As name for a structural relation, the unity of religion and dance itself appears as one phenomenon, one moment in a fabric of structural relations comprised itself as well of these four other possibilities. "Unity of religion and dance" represents one family of features—one that van der Leeuw is able to perceive by virtue of its difference from the conceptual nets described in this chapter. At the same time, in so far as the conceptual net naming the unity of religion and dance identifies dance as enacting a *unity of life,* then this first concept necessarily plays a role in interpreting the significance of other historical moments where dance and religion do not appear in the same guise. In other words, the four other conceptual nets described here appear as structural derivatives of the spiraling rhythm between image and movement, reason and experience, which the concept of dance as enacting the unity of life predicts. In so far as van der Leeuw succeeds in comprehending instances of dance by way of the other patterns he identifies, he demonstrates the value of his first phenomenological structure—regardless of whether or not such a moment ever really existed in history. The four other relational possibilities between dance and religion that Van der Leeuw recreates are: transition, antithesis, influences, and harmony.

This chapter introduces these four conceptual structures and assesses their implications for scholars in religious studies. In short, in identifying these structural relations, van der Leeuw rejects the idea that a unity of religion and dance is ever possible, in practice or in theory. He animates the differences among the various structural relations in order to argue that there is no moment of recognizing a phenomenon as either dance or religion in which that recognition does not presuppose both the inevitability and the incomprehensibility of their simultaneous appearance. In a conclusion to Part 2, I continue the argument begun at the end of Chapter 8, providing a phenomenological defense for the study of dance in and as religion.

TRANSITION

The first of the four remaining structural relations van der Leeuw outlines is "breakup of unity" or "transition" (S 36; W 44). Next to the unity of dance and religion, this conceptual net is most important because transition represents the perspective on religion and dance capable of seeing other shapes of the relationship as possibilities. It represents the perspective of van der Leeuw himself as a phenomenologist in modern society. As van der Leeuw notes, for a person who perceives dance and religion as comprising a unity, the question of their relationship, of possible "paths and boundaries" between them, does not arise. A given instance of dancing may appear as "prayer, work, and dance" at once (S 16; W 33). By contrast, the fact that the question of *relationship* arises for him is a sign that he is *between*. In his historical study of religions, he notices coincidences of religion and dance, but he does so because they strike him as strange. He does not live in a society where such perspectives of unity are common—quite the reverse.

As van der Leeuw employs his phenomenological method to recreate imaginatively the forms in which this strangeness appears to him, a new structural relation comes into view—"transition." It represents a new perspective on his own context. He becomes conscious of how his perceptions of religion and dance are constituted by his movement between the kinds of moments he inhabits and those he studies. Van der Leeuw elaborates: "We find ourselves, so to speak, always in transition [*in een overgang*] from the primitive sphere of magical continuity to the differentiated sphere of the 'modern' spirit [*geeste*], a transition which is eternal [*eeuwig*], because it is determined not temporally, but structurally" (S 267; W 440-1). The "we" here includes those for whom "paths and boundaries" between religion and dance appear as a concern. For such people, to be "always in transition" is to be moving, yet not on the way to somewhere else in time or in space. As a *structure*, transition is "eternal." As discussed in Chapter 6, to be a phenomenologist is to cultivate this movement among historical moments as comprising a *perspective* from which to view any conception of the relationship of religion and dance that presents itself as "true." It is a phenomenologist's movement (his being in transition) that allows him to affirm any appearance of religion and dance in its historical particularity (whether it appears as "magical continuity" or "differentiated spheres") as internally related to the structural possibilities it excludes.

Examining his own culture through the lens of this structure, van der Leeuw discerns two other signs of transition (besides his own project): a desire to make "religious dance" and an unacknowledged use of rhythmic movement as a medium of cultural expression. He identifies both as "relics" or "fossils" of living dance (van der Leeuw uses the terms *overblijfsel*—"remainder, remnant" [S 39; W 49]—and *survival* [S 36; W 46]): such phenomena imply but do not realize an awareness of the religious potency of dance.[1]

Regarding the first, van der Leeuw claims that those who aspire to make "sacred" or "religious dances" in contrast to "profane" dances express their belief in an inherent opposition between religion and dance, even as they profess to overcome it. In so far as such persons aspire to standards of "external continuity" that ensure that their dancing will be a special brand of dance, they define the religious component of a dance as accidental to the dancing itself. A dance, for example, appears as religion if it conforms to certain rules in the choice of subject matter, aesthetic forms, performing venues, costumes, intent, etc. Retronyms such as "religious dance" arise to name that subset of forms which succeeds in becoming something more than just plain dance. In van der Leeuw's reading, this desire for religious dancing both acknowledges that dance can conduct experiences of power *and* confirms that religion and dance are discrete activities needing mediation. It is a desire, he observes, that tends to gather interest among a select few in society who seek to elevate the art in the eyes of a larger public (S 36; W 45).

By interpreting this yearning for religious dance as a "relic," that is, from the perspective provided by his phenomenological understanding of dance as enacting the unity of life, van der Leeuw hones in on a contradiction that suggests why such projects have yet to revolutionize the study or practice of dance and religion. Such appeals represent an appreciation for what dancing can be in terms of a longing for what dance no longer is (regardless of what it actually was). Where the distinction between sacred and profane, or religion and dance, is presumed as the condition for making religious dance, then the distinction cannot be overcome.[2] A dance made to be religious loses claim to being "its own articulation"; its meaning is dictated by verbal, doctrinal expressions of faith and religion.

Van der Leeuw's analysis here applies to scholars of religion seeking to study dance as well in a way that aligns with the conclusions of Part 1. A scholar who predicates her study of religion and dance on a distinction between objective scholarship and theology cannot perceive "beautiful movement" *in itself* as a conduit for power. When the intent to appreciate a relationship is founded on an assumption of antithesis, then "dance" appears as "religion" only in so far as it meets the standards of scholarly accountablity established on the model of texts.

Van der Leeuw's second example of transition carries further implications. Van der Leeuw finds signs of transition in the parades and processions that accompany "solemn moments and in representative events," whether funerals, marriages, graduation ceremonies, military functions, dance halls, and in general, the practices of love and war (S 43; W 54). Without being aware of it, van der Leeuw argues, citizens of modern cultures express "a need to make life rhythmical" (S 37; W 46). As he continues: "When something matters in life, one feels festive; the expression of life becomes stylized into a fixed, rhythmical form. We still cannot tear ourselves loose from the compulsive fascination of a squad of marching soldiers, even without music. It awakens in us a vague feeling of the rhythm of life, the festively moving background of all existence. Every event needs a rhythm" (S 37; W 46).

Applying his phenomenological analysis to such forms, van der Leeuw discerns an opposite trajectory to the one represented by the desire for religious dancing. In this case, the unity of religion and dance is assumed, through repressed. The fact that citizens of the modern world repeat such movements, van der Leeuw avers, cannot be explained in relation to rational goals; "not a single argument is advanced" (S 42; W 53). Rather, citizens participate in such movements for the experience itself—the experience of a compelling power, one that stirs, meets, and guides the energies of those involved. Van der Leeuw remarks that "power issues" from the "innumerable demonstrations, meetings, witnesses, to which our social and political differences give rise":"'Something' is present which can[not] be represented: a supra-individual power which constrains free movement [*vrije bewegingen*]" (S 42; W 52-53). When these phenomena are understood as special forms of religion and dance, van der Leeuw explains, the mystery clears. Although the movement is monotonous and counterpoint is absent (S 43; W 53), the rhythm drives a spiral of discovery and response through a logic of bodily becoming. As people notice and submit themselves to the rhythmic patterns, they find within themselves the capacity to make the movements. As they lose themselves in the performance of those movements, they feel power—the radiating power of mastery, the filling power of being danced—as a function of how they are constraining their own movements. As they act, they make real the vision of the world that those movements represent. In this sense, such movements betray consciousness of phenomenological links between religion and dance described in Chapter 8.

Continuing with his analysis, van der Leeuw concludes that neither of these examples of transition is either dance "in the full sense of the word" or religion; they represent "petrified" dance (S 43; W 53). What is missing in both cases is the ingredient mentioned at the end of Chapter 8: a *consciousness* of dance as enacting a unity of life. Such a consciousness provides the context within which it is possible to appreciate any instance of dance as a phenomenon, as one manifestation of a larger rhythm. "No matter how many relics it has preserved in its structure and connected phenomena," van der Leeuw implies, a dance cannot be studied, watched, or performed as art or religion unless participants have this consciousness (S 49; W 62). People—scholars included—may still dance dances whose names refer to mimetic and ecstatic forms of dance, such as the fox trot and the pavane (peacock dance), or the tarantella and Morris dancing; they may enjoy forms of dance in music and in children's games. However, where people are educated to believe that any relation between dance and religion is *external* and thus accidental to the practice of either, then there is little motivation to create either aesthetic forms or theoretical categories capable of realizing the religious potency of dance. We need both.

CONFLICT BETWEEN DANCE AND RELIGION

Van der Leeuw's application of his phenomenological analysis to signs of transition brings into view another structural relation—the second pole in relation to which a person in "transition" finds himself suspended, namely a state of antithesis, "Enmity between Dance and Religion" (S 50; W 63). In the instances that comprise this fabric of particulars, a given culture, group, or individual perceives dance and religion as enemies. In seeking to recreate the forms in which enmity occurs, van der Leeuw identifies a pattern: people perceive dance and religion as enemies where they perceive the act of dancing as exercising human attention and energies away from the goals or experiences they associate with the name "religion." While conflict between dance and religion is "ancient," van der Leeuw explains, it finds "its most relentless form in the late Middle Ages," a form carried on in Protestant Christian polemics (S 50; W 63). As van der Leeuw notes, "Protestant churches in general are not favorably inclined toward the dance, and the idea of a religious dance is inconceivable to them" (S 51; W 63). For van der Leeuw this enmity is the distinctive mark of a "modern" society; as he insists, to be "modern" is to take this conflict for granted as given.[3] Such is the preponderance of Christian examples in this section that a better title is perhaps "Enmity between Dance and Christianity."

In imaginatively recreating the motivations impelling such hostility, van der Leeuw gives priority to two cultural alliances as condemning dance in the eyes of "the Church": "the connection between the dance and the theater" and—a "second, deeper reason"—the "close connection between dance and eroticism" (S 53-4; W 66, 68). For example, he explains how early Christians living amidst Greco-Roman culture repudiated "heathen theater." Theater was featured in "pagan" religions and linked with the kinds of world-oriented activities early Christians suspected. Dance suffered by association. Van der Leeuw concludes:

The opposition of the Christian Church to the theater has grounds which are basically historical . . . We do not see theater and religion, but two different religions, one against the another: the ancient fertility religion of the *sacer ludus,* with its candor and secular symbols, and the new ascetic religion of Christendom. The theater must pay for its fidelity to the ancient primitive religious forms [*oude, primitief-religieuze vormen*] with the hostility of the new religions. (S 97; W 132)

As scholars have noted, in forging a Christian identity, early Christians appropriated many aspects of pagan religion even as they discounted others. Dance was one of the casualties, falling to the side of the pagan.[4] Yet by making the point that the early Church opposed dance because members of another religion were practicing it, van der Leeuw interprets Christian hostility to dance as expressing a recognition that dancing was (and can be) a medium of religious experience and expression.

In van der Leeuw's account, a second and related factor of Christian enmity towards dance was and remains the association of dance with eroticism. As van der Leeuw confirms, the dance "even the simplest and most proper, brings out the glory of the body; and even in its most innocent form it serves for the mutual attraction of the sexes" (S 54; W 68). His analysis here parallels his analysis of the relation between dance and theater: he interprets Christian antipathy towards dance as a function of its opposition to another religion. Here, Christian opposition to dance is mediated by a conception of the body borrowed from Neoplatonic philosophy. Christian apologists, van der Leeuw relates, "took over from the Greeks, along with the idea of the divinity and immortality of the soul, the idea of the evil of the body."[5] As he reasons:

It is obvious that a view of life which shrinks from the body cannot stand for [*dulden*—bear, suffer] beautiful movement; that a religion which exalts virginity above all else must hate the enticements of the moving body; that the hope for release from the body of this death expects no benefit from expression of [any] feeling, and certainly not from any expression of the holy, through dance. (S 54-5; W 68-9)

Here, van der Leeuw mobilizes his phenomenological approach to affirm and critique Christian enmity toward dance. On the one hand, he affirms such enmity as one possible manifestation of a relationship between religion and dance—one given in the idea of dance as enacting a unity of life. On the other, he exposes this position as contradicting itself: the need for the hostility bears witness to historical and phenomenological links between religion and dance that the hostility arises to deny. In his view, it is this self-contradicting strand of Christian thinking that "has been the out-spoken enemy of the body and all sensual pleasures, which it never considers innocent" (S 55; W 69).

Several implications for scholars of religious studies follow from van der Leeuw's descriptions of Christian enmity towards dance. The first and obvious point is that any instance of hostility towards dance must be interpreted as testifying to what it denies—the ability of dance to enact a unity of life. Hostility would not be necessary if antithesis did not need to be created and enforced. In other words, in so far as enmity towards dance is perceived as protecting the sacrality of a given religion from the corrupting influence of culture, by implication, dance has the power to threaten religion, to contaminate the sacred. Dance appears in the condemnation of it as a competing religion. Van der Leeuw's conclusion is ingenious: the impetus driving antithesis to dance (in Christianity at least) is not an anti-theater, anti-body or anti-sexuality attitude per se, but the acknowledgement of dance, structurally speaking, as capable of enacting the logic of bodily becoming, the spiral of culture, and their interdependent unity, and thus giving meaning to bodies and sexuality other than those desired by the Church.

Van der Leeuw's analysis of antithesis also illuminates the theories of religion discussed in Chapters 1 through 4. As noted, theories and methods of religion imbued with modern consciousness express the structure of antithesis; they assume the opposition of religion and dance. Yet in doing so, they adopt as true a theological evaluation of dance based on an historical moment of conflict between "two religions." From this perspective, the absence of dance from theory and method in the study of religion appears as evidence for historical and phenomenological coincidences of religion and dance. The primary obstacle to considering dance as religion, then, does not appear as a function of theological bias (requiring redoubled adherence to an emergence narrative of the field), but rather as a function of the belief that the practice of writing exercises the capacity of reason to free itself from determination by experience—one's own or that of others. This belief in writing drives and expresses one moment of the paradox of expression—the one in which images arrest movement. As van der Leeuw's analysis in Chapter 8 suggests, the problem for scholars of religion interested in dance is not writing per se, but an inability to perceive their writing as itself a kind of dancing—as a mode of participating in a paradox of expression common to both writing and dancing. In Western scholarship, at least since Descartes, the authority of writing in relation to theology is founded on one of the dangers of representation van der Leeuw identifies: fixing images to the point of denying the movement that enables those images to mean or communicate.

At the same time, however, van der Leeuw's interpretation of his history illuminates a path forward. Antithesis is not an end point. Once disclosed as an antithesis, the very disclosure foreshadows the dissolution of that antithesis given the phenomenological structure of dance. Van der Leeuw sees signs of this turn in his time. For one, modern social organization, while demanding the exclusion of dance from the realms of religion and art, creates a situation in which a few self-selected people focus on dancing as their art of choice and begin to explore its peculiar expressive potential. The isolation of dance as one moment of culture can enable a growing appreciation of dancing in relation to other activities. Likewise, as van der Leeuw asserts, the "modern" isolation of the body from the soul or reason forces a reconception of what it means to be human. While the same framework of antithesis remains intact, people are turning it upside down, elevating the body over and against reason. Describing what he calls the "cult of the body" (S 55; W 69), van der Leeuw writes:

> I do not hesitate to greet it as desirable that the body is no longer considered a negligible quantity . . . we shall not go far astray if we see, in the continually growing demands which things of the body make upon our culture, an expression of the same spirit which in psychology and philosophy, once more desires to view man as a unity; not as a soul in an accidental body, but as a single organism whose deepest essence expresses itself as much in the least movement of the body as in speech or thought. We have thereby gradually reconquered for ourselves the possibility of expression through bodily movement. (S 56; W 70)

As van der Leeuw explains, these reversals in attitude and intent are *predicted* by his phenomenological account of dance as enacting a unity of life. The rhythms embedded in this account predict dance's own disappearance (in the images of modern thought), its rebirth (in aesthetic forms), and the necessary cooperation of both of these moments in the process of raising people's consciousness of the potency of dance as art and religion, enacting unities of life.

Wrenched from bodies and fixed in verbal images, dance stands revealed and concealed. Yet the phenomenological structure of dance suggests that even the most extreme cases of this wrenching—where societies succeed in denying any obvious role to bodily becoming as a form of religion—represent the far swing of a pendulum. In the form of an image, however maligned, dance is both dead and alive, filling out, in its dead form, a dialectical spiral constitutive of culture. Van der Leeuw urges his readers to remember that every act of dancing contains the seeds of its own negation in an image, and that every image of dance contains the seeds of its negation in the creation of new dance forms. As he insists, "history is never finished with anything. Before *lavolta* is finished, the movement of the dance reverses" (S 35; W 32).

Thus, for scholars interested in studying religion and dance, the task is clear. By articulating the distinctions that mediate moments of enmity between religion and dance (body versus mind, or reason versus experience), scholars create opportunities for perceiving those oppositions as one phase of an underlying rhythm. Scholars thereby not only help to rehabilitate consciousness of dance as an expression of life (as described in Chapter 8), they defuse the theological bias against dance by disclosing the historical and phenomenological roots of that bias; they defuse the antitheological biases against dance by exposing writing as disciplinary practice, structurally linked with dance through participation in the paradox of expression. In short, scholars *can* dismantle obstacles in the field to acknowledge dance as a medium of religious experience and expression and they *must* do so in pursuing the goal of critical, empathetic understanding of religion.

MOMENTE

Further applying his phenomenological account of dance as enacting the unity of life, van der Leeuw identifies a third structural relation— *momente*. The English translation of *momente* as "influences" implies an external relationship that van der Leeuw, as noted above, patently rejects. His argument here is not that there are moments in history where people perceive dance as meaningful due to its influence on religion, or vice versa. Rather, he uses this term to recreate and understand the conditions that give rise to divergent perceptions of dance and religion within any one religious tradition. As is the case for all world religions, some voices within a tradition may forbid dancing and others welcome it. In such cases, coincidences of religion and dance are mediated not by a general appreciation of dance as enacting a unity of life, or by a set of criteria external to the dance or by a perception of antithesis. Particulars appearing in the fabric of "moments" share this feature: they isolate one facet of dancing over and against others as the conduit of its religious quality. Discerning the meaning of such moments, van der Leeuw insists, requires that a scholar proceed "atomistically," discussing points in history across traditions where "religion and the dance touch and interpenetrate" (S 47; W 72).

Given this definition, it is not surprising that van der Leeuw's naming of such moments hews closely to the styles of dance as culture discussed in Chapter 8—striding, hovering, and walking. As described in Chapter 8, each style articulates one dimension of how and why dance may be perceived as enacting the unity of life. Each style appears as the defining feature of a dance form to the exclusion of the other styles. The cases van der Leeuw uses to illustrate the two structures (unity and moments) overlap, again undercutting any sense of chronological relation among his structures. The three "moments" he names, with allusion to Nietzsche, are the Apollonian, the Dionysian, and the Human. A brief description of each follows.

In recreating the phenomenological form of moments that appear as Apollonian, van der Leeuw engages the style of mimetic dances, striding for mastery:

> Apollonian movement is, above all, order, which calms the soul and fills it with quiet . . . The movement of the rhythm awakens the awareness of a background to life, a cosmic order which extends this life to its limits [*grens*], where it has no purpose other than through and in that which is beyond, the holy [*het Heilige*]. (S 60-61; W 76-7)

Within Greek religions, Apollo dances. The act of making and/or watching the rhythmic movements associated with him draws the

dancer into an awareness of a "cosmos"—a larger order encompassing the given of her own world, in relation to which her life attains
purpose. The unfathomable background to her life appears in and
through the movement as a power that is both inaccessible and
nonetheless assured: "Everything dark, everything ecstatic, everything intoxicated and disintegrating, everything infinite and unac-
countable is excluded" in order to make apparent (as in the music of
Bach) a "shining world of fine lines which cross and then diverge,
drawing us inescapably and yet filling us with awe" (S 61; W 78). In
such moments, van der Leeuw explains, dance appears as religion for
the way in which it appears to participate in the creation and realization of the cosmos—the seizing of life.

In contrast to the "restrained and ordered" Apollonian movement,
van der Leeuw describes a second kind of moment in which dances
draw forth the ecstatic potency of dance as religion, such as the
"raving dance of the dervishes and maenads" (S 61; W 79):

> The dervishes dance until they have forgotten everything.
> Earthly, bodily life is discarded, blown away. Dancing is not a
> secular pastime, but training for blessedness. In ecstasy, the
> body becomes light and the chains of the soul loosen . . . The
> personality is lost in the whirlwind, while the narrow confines
> of the body and the environment are extended to infinity. (S 62;
> W 80, 82)

Commenting on this example, he concludes: "It is thus not aston-
ishing that the dance belongs to the technical apparatus of many
types of mysticism" (S 62; W 82). These forms of dancing develop the
style of hovering to the exclusion of striding: rhythmic movement is
performed to dissolve the sensible boundaries through which humans
negotiate time and space, self and other, extending them to infinity. In
such cases, people embrace dance for its ability to effect this sensory
openness—to facilitate experiences in which the "depths [of life]
become visible and its undertones audible" (S 60; W 77). As particulars

comprising this structural relation, van der Leeuw cites, in addition to the Sufi dervishes, the Quakers, Hebrew Bible accounts of Saul and David, and Hellenic plays—all moments in life of Islamic, Christian and Greek religions respectively where members embrace dance for this ecstatic potency. As van der Leeuw notes, the "Quakers received their name from the peculiar spasmodic shaking which seizes the pious at the moment of illumination" (S 62, W 82). In this regard, he could have mentioned the Shakers as well. While the Quakers went on to develop a practice of silent worship, the Shakers developed a strong dance tradition. However, the Shaker dance history is marked by periods of both ordered line and pattern dances as well as the more ecstatic spontaneous dances he is describing here. See Andrews (1940) and (1953).

The third "moment" of dance that van der Leeuw adds to his account is one he describes as "the human." "The human" represents instances of dance whose meaning people perceive as a function of his very first statement about dance: that all one needs to dance is a human body. In the act of dancing, dancers and spectators experience more than is actually presented in the story or steps of a given dance itself; they enjoy a visceral experience of their own embodied capacity for creative expression. Drawing upon his phenomenological structures to grasp the meaning of such appearances, van der Leeuw explains how dance facilitates this experience: it makes visible the logic of bodily becoming as the "background" or rhythm of life. To be a body is to move; to move is to bring new shapes of life into being; to bring new shapes of life into being is to create. By revealing the body as the locus of its own becoming, dance reveals humans as participants in and vehicles of the rhythm of life.

While van der Leeuw's account of this third moment is admittedly brief and vague, it serves a purpose in his project by laying the groundwork for a philosophy of religion and dance. He closes this section of the text with a long quotation by Emil Utitz that gestures towards a metaphysics of dance. He quotes:

"Through the shaping power of art we experience that humanity genuine and unfalsified, as we experience the beauty of a dancer in her dance. As long as we are concerned with this type, she dances her beauty. Not just to put it vainly on display; no, because only through this process does she express her essence, and always more purely, more fully, the better the shaping succeeds. Here, within art, the human discovers the most difficult test of its capacity to bear weight; for it [the human] does not appear before us 'in' various roles, nor only in work 'on' a work of art. No; it must assert itself through itself."[6]

Here, a person dancing expresses the essence of (her) humanity. In this presentation, paradoxes prevail. What "we" experience as "genuine and unfalsified" in the dancer's dance *is* the "shaping power of art." In dancing she "expresses her essence" as she reveals herself to be a *process* of becoming her self through this shaping power. The better she "shapes" her art, the more her "humanity"—that is, her power to shape—appears as "genuine." Thus, what appears so revealed in her dance is humanity as a process of shaping and asserting "itself through itself." What appears in her dance is a logic of bodily becoming, proceeding through a culture spiral of discovery and response. There is no universal "essence" at all. The "genuine" is a function of an individual's art, her process of making images of herself as image maker. Dance reveals this self-doubling action by concealing it in the singular form of an individual making a simple gesture.

Thus, in embracing the capacity of dance to make apparent "the human," van der Leeuw introduces *dancing* as a resource for knowing and articulating something distinctive about what it means to be human. As van der Leeuw suggests: "Any expression of the divine through the human is, naturally, in a very special sense the prior right of the dance. The movement of the body often expresses more of the totality and the background of life than words or sounds are able to do" (S 66; W 88). What stands revealed as "divine" in and through the dance is a logic of bodily becoming that cannot be arrested in image or word because it enables both. When van der Leeuw concludes that "the maternal, founding movement of all life is the dance" (S 65; W 81, my translation), his point is phenomenologically based. Structurally speaking, dance appears to van der Leeuw as an activity that is and represents the process by which humans give birth to the meaning of their humanity, their bodily being on earth.

In offering his analysis of "moments," then, van der Leeuw provides scholars of religion with conceptual tools for delivering a critical affirmation of religion, and for doing so in relation to the act of dancing. He appreciates the appearance of such "moments" to him as a function of both the particular religious context of that moment and his phenomenological practice. On one hand, he can *affirm* the meaning, for example, that a dance of ecstatic self-loss appears to have for those within a tradition who do it: "The movement releases power, dissipates it, so to speak, and empties the soul so that it may be filled with the god" (S 65; W 79). On the other, he can provide a *critical* perspective on that meaning based on his phenomenological account of dance as religion: "at the same time life is grasped and ruled... Rhythm which has become independent leads to the rhythm of life itself" (S 65; W 80). While he refrains from judging whether or not a tradition's claims to god's filling are or can be realized, he can explain this perception of truth as a *function* of performing *rhythmic bodily movement*. Van der Leeuw is able to affirm dance as a moment of religion as well as reflect critically on its meaning by investigating the ways in which it stylizes a field of phenomenological possibilities evident across traditions. His structures thus provide him with interpretive webs whose strands are ever stretched, pulled, and rewoven by the weight of particular appearances of dance and religion.

HARMONY

Although the preceding patterns of identity and difference might seem to exhaust the spectrum of possible relationships appearing in history between dance and religion, van der Leeuw offers one more: "harmony." "It is possible for beauty and holiness to interpenetrate so that one must speak of a harmony" (S 67; W 89). Here, the coincidence of religion and dance is not mediated by the contexts of cultural life, external criteria (as in transition), a mutual antipathy (as in modern consciousness), or by isolating and developing one vector of dance as enacting the unity of cultural and bodily life (as for the moments). In these instances, people perceive experiences of beauty and power as "interpenetrating" fruits of a particular form of dance itself. In such cases, the ordered articulation of the body effects an experience of communication with a rhythmic becoming—the background—of life. Citing examples from "Indian dances" of Java, Bali, and "Indo-China," van der Leeuw explains:

> Every nuance of spreading the fingers and moving the arms becomes so much an expression of the movement of the soul, and every movement of the soul is so much a step in the great progress of man to, from, and in God, that we must speak of a complete harmony ... anyone who has ever watched Indian dancing senses that here the inner movement of the mystic ascent [*mystieken opgang*] of the soul to God [*in God*] has become visible. The body has completely become an instrument. (S 67; W 89-90)

This passage is troubling to scholars. Van der Leeuw hazards an interpretation of Indian dances by invoking Western theological language, referring to soul and God and mystical ascent. Nevertheless, another reading is possible. Van der Leeuw is tracing the unraveling edge of his own phenomenological nets. Just prior to this passage, van der Leeuw refers his readers to a "specialist" in Indian religions, acknowledging his own ignorance of Indian dance and his need for correction by historians of religion. Then, in an attempt to recreate imaginatively the meaning that these dances have for those who do them or who watch them, he appeals to the experience of dancing he aims to study. The implication is that his readers must themselves engage in the practice of phenomenology in order to flesh out and understand the conditions enabling such appearances of harmony. The best he can do is acknowledge that the dance *is* religion; it is the medium in and through which people not only express a sense of their bodily participation in power, but actually come to know what appears to them in their dance as what is.

Thus, van der Leeuw uses this final structure not only to communicate to readers the extent of their and his lack of understanding, but to pinpoint its cause. "We" have not learned to relate to our bodies as "instruments." We have not learned to discipline ourselves to the form and rhythms of our bodies as the medium for religious experience and expression. Until we do, we will have difficulty understanding moments in religious life characterized by this kind of "harmony." In the West, van der Leeuw contends, we do not find this harmony "except in heaven" (S 67; W 90). In his posthumous edition, Smelik qualifies van der Leeuw's more radical critique, adding, "or in what the mind has reached in literature, in music, and in painting" (S 67).

Conclusion to Part Two
Can Dance Be Religion?

For scholars interested in the study of dance and religion, van der Leeuw's phenomenological method, his theory of religion, and his five structures characterizing appearances of religion and dance provide a rich if challenging inheritance. To sift through the value of this work and some of its implications, I revisit the question van der Leeuw poses at the beginning of *Sacred and Profane Beauty*. He asks: Can dance be a holy act? Is dance something for which scholars of religion should develop theoretical and methodological approaches?

At first glance, it seems that van der Leeuw would respond with a hearty "Yes!" He identifies numerous instances in which something appears to him as appearing to someone as having meaning as both religion and dance—as beautiful movement and an expression of dislocating power. Such moments, he implies, demand attention for what they tell scholars about *religion* and not only about *dance*.

On second glance, however, van der Leeuw seems less optimistic. He rejects the idea that any general theory of such moments is possible. Such coincidences arise as singular events occurring in a complex, multi-layered relationship between a phenomenologist and that which appears. Any coincidence of dance and religion represents an *appearance* of *meaning*. It will not appear in the form of a historical fact, nor in the form of a dogmatic judgment; it will and can appear only as a moment in the lived experience of an individual person who is open to such a possibility. Given this singularity, van der Leeuw suggests that it is impossible to derive any stable account of when or why a coincidence of religion and dance appears.

Moreover, as van der Leeuw insists, any moment of unity that does appear is itself fragmentary and ephemeral. A coincidence of religion and dance appears only to someone who perceives the relationship between religion and dance as a problem in the first place—someone in transition, someone raised and educated to perceive of dance and religion as occupying conflicting spheres of human life. It appears only to a person educated to believe in reading and writing. Correlatively, any appearance of unity is always already a moment in the web of structural relations that enable "unity" to appear—a web that includes the shapes of transition, enmity, moments, harmony, etc. The degree to which this situation holds for dance in contrast to other moments of cultural life is distinct because, as van der Leeuw notes, dance is the art that has suffered most at the hands of Christian and Western authorities. Drama, visual art, architecture, music, poetry, and literature have never experienced the degree and range of antipathy that dancing has. Only dance fills out all five of van der Leeuw's structures.

Even so, the fact that dance has suffered so, ironically enough, van der Leeuw interprets as evidence of his point that phenomenologically speaking, every act of dancing, in so far as its medium is bodily movement, enacts and expresses a unity of life. How that "unity" is conceived, composed, inflected, and interpreted is different and fleeting in every case. Yet dance inevitably animates the relatedness of dimensions of life that "religion" works to distinguish as sacred and profane: the body that will be resurrected can prance seductively. Resistance by religious authorities to dancing implies that dancing represents a threat to their ability to distinguish "religion" from the rest of life as a "last word." This diagnosis carries a paradoxical implication: only by crafting theories that insist upon an irreconcilable difference between dance and religion can scholars guarantee the possibility that they will be able to perceive the coincidence of religion and dance. What distinguishes dance from religion is its ability to enact a unity of bodily and cultural life that extends to include all moments of "religion" and "dance."

Summarizing with regard to art in general, van der Leeuw writes, a "complete unity of religion and art is neither conceivable nor desirable" (S 332; W 460). It is not conceivable because concepts of unity and disunity arise hand in hand; it is not desirable because such a unity would deny the difference between religion and art that enables art to serve as a critical perspective on the study and practice of religion—especially in its consciousness of dance. When a coincidence does appear, it does so only as a "disconcerting miracle": "It does not pay to strive for it, for we do not attain it. It is granted us as a rare, disconcerting miracle" (S 271).

In van der Leeuw's schema, then, the study of dance in and as religion appears as equally necessary and impossible. How are we to proceed? How are we to negotiate a "disconcerting miracle"? How can we affirm an historical case that appears as both religion and dance in a way that honors the difference between religion and dance as the necessary condition for their independent vitality?

PATHS AND BOUNDARIES

Van der Leeuw starts us along a path towards an answer by providing us with provisions for the journey. A brief review of five points is helpful for plotting a future course.

First, van der Leeuw underlines the importance of remembering that religion and dance are *phenomena*—that is, *names* for the *structural relations* that someone identifies as enabling her to perceive something as having meaning for someone by virtue of its relation to other moments appearing to her under the same name. As names, religion and dance are human constructions that function as *ideal types;* they are normative classifications that humans project upon the rich manifold of what is. Names conceal what they intend to reveal; they impose order where there is none, and only in this way do they enable intelligibility. At the same time, these "constructions" are *given* to an observer: they dawn upon her when something appears. Thus, scholars must remember that religion and dance are *phenomena* in this van der Leeuwian sense so that they only not maintain a healthy suspicion of any definition of religion, dance, or their relationship, but so that they also take responsibility for their role in the life of those definitions and work to cultivate an ongoing receptivity to further appearances of their meaning.

Second, van der Leeuw offers scholars guidance in how to participate in this ongoing process of receiving and recreating forms of life that appear to be both religion and dance. Any methodological approach must be phenomenological in the sense he describes—indirect, dynamic, and holistic. A scholar must cultivate vulnerability to appearances of dance and religion by employing imaginative empathy, suspending judgment, and opening himself and his findings to constant correction by historical facts and theological claims. In short, a scholar interested in acknowledging dance as religion must learn to sustain within himself a tension between the need to arrest movement in images and the desire to dissolve images into a rhythmic flow of experience, between the need to generate a rational explanation of rhythmic bodily movement and the need to acknowledge it as much as possible on its own terms. He must be able to "bear and work with the tension which has been created" and love the crooked path (S 283; W 270).

Only a phenomenological approach of this kind can serve to dislodge the primary obstacles that have foreclosed scholarly attention to dance to date—namely, theological bias against dance and scholarly bias against theology. By moving between the historical record and theological commitments (including his own) as his phenomenological method allows, van der Leeuw does so. He finds support in challenging both the phenomenological assumptions of his theological tradition and the theological assumptions lodged within historical accounts of "religion." He interprets Christian hostility towards dance as evidence of what he finds in other cultures: that dance is and can be an expression of life. He honors his own theological commitments to the paradoxical forms of God's (dis)appearing by attending to those aspects of (non-Christian) religious life that elude the grasp of scholarly writing. That he finds dance as religion in the process should come as no surprise for those familiar with the narrative of generative tension relayed in Part 1. In defusing the antitheology polemics that have characterized the field, van der Leeuw makes room for rethinking the privilege accorded to writing as the medium for pursuing, representing, and authorizing true and certain knowledge.

Third, as the previous points imply, practice of a phenomenological method like van der Leeuw's produces the fruits that it does only when a scholar consciously and critically engages her living life as the enabling condition of her understanding. As van der Leeuw insists, understanding is a full-bodied action. Van der Leeuw acknowledges that it is impossible for scholars of religious studies to discard their subjectivity or their individual humanity in pursuit of facts. Such a concept of "objectivity" may work for other disciplines studying other kinds of phenomena. However, in so far as religion as a phenomenon represents an *appearance* of *meaning*, then the living life of the scholar is integral to the process of scholarship. For a scholar of religious studies, the difference between two pieces of wood nailed together and a cross is the problem. While it may be a fact that someone perceives those pieces as a cross, it is not a fact that that wood *is* a cross. To be a cross is to have meaning for someone as a cross. A historian who calls the wood a cross makes a theological assumption. At that same time, the meaning of the wood as cross is not necessarily a function of what someone *believes*. Meaning is physical, emotional, kinetic, and may be intellectual; it appears in how people think, feel, and move in relation to what appears to them. Given this "object" of study, the most direct method for apprehending the meaning that something has for someone may be to recreate imaginatively the sensory experience of that person based on the signs left behind. For such imaginative acts, as described in Chapter 6, the stuff of one's own experiences is the material out of which the recreations in their emotional, physical richness can be made.

At the same time, van der Leeuw admits that it is impossible to experience what another person experiences. It is even impossible to re-experience one's own past experiences. We have no access to any primal or immediate experience. Even if a scholar is or were to become an adherent to the tradition he studies, he still would not experience what someone else who identifies herself as belonging to the tradition does. Conversely, even when a scholar insists on maintaining a healthy distance from a tradition, he cannot help working out of his own matrix of irretrievable experiences. With this perspective, van der Leeuw defuses debates over whether someone inside or outside a tradition has a better view. Neither group has a pure experience of "it." Far-flung outsiders who study a tradition are as much a part of its life as insiders seeking to defend the distinctiveness of what they do as "religion."

In affirming understanding as a full-bodied action, van der Leeuw also opens the door to a radical idea: namely, that the act of *learning to dance* might be as important to a scholar in his study of religion as are the acts of learning to read and write. To learn to dance is to develop the physical consciousness required to notice movement patterns and recreate them in one's own movement. If what must be understood is meaning as described above, then perhaps learning the movement patterns characteristic of a given religious tradition can be as illuminating and as critical an activity as learning its verbal forms. The objectivity in this case is given in the attention and discipline required to develop the ability to recreate for himself the kinetic images in which another's experiences appear to him as having meaning. A trained physical consciousness affords a critical perspective in a manner similar to the practice of reading and writing: by exercising a given set of human capabilities as a locus of discovery and response. Where the act of writing exercises an ability to imagine I have no body, the act of dancing exercises a kinetic imagination. Where the act of writing may guide those who practice it to perceive texts, beliefs, and literary forms as vehicles of knowledge, the act of dancing may guide those who practice it to attend to bodily movements, gestures, and kinetic images as vehicles of knowledge. While writing may always retain a privilege in scholarly circles as a primary means for the collection and dissemination of information, van der Leeuw's project suggests that the ability of writing to accomplish such tasks may depend in part upon whether those who write also dance, or for that matter, draw, sing, play, or build. Such aesthetic practices can provide a perspective from which to reflect upon the strengths and limitations of writing itself as a bodily practice.

Fourth, not only does van der Leeuw orient scholars in how to think about theory, method, and their own lived participation in the study of phenomena, he offers his own definitions of religion and dance which, while not the only, inevitable, or definitive fruits of his phenomenological practice, are nevertheless helpful in generating further studies of religion and dance. Van der Leeuw's theory of religion as an expression of power is a case in point. His dynamic definition of religion not only encourages scholars of religion to look again at instances of dancing that earlier scholars dismiss as unimportant to their studies, he does so with the intention of discerning how these instances trouble illusions of verbal mastery recreated among scholars themselves—even and especially where they employ that mastery in articulating their own limits. By claiming that humans exist in and through acts of communication they themselves enable, van der Leeuw opens a critical perspective on how the definitions of religion reproduce the life condition of the scholars who deploy them.

The names van der Leeuw generates for the structural relations defining coincidences of religion and dance are also helpful, especially when understood in the context of his phenomenological approach.

These names—unity, transition, enmity, moments, and harmony—do not represent discrete, historical categories into which to fit facts. Nor do they plot an evolutionary path. As categories they are interdependent, arising at once as a nexus of conflicting perspectives. Any one case of rhythmic bodily movement may demonstrate aspects of more than one structural relation. The value of these terms, then, lies not in their *actuality*, but in their *potentiality*: their ability to allow a scholar to perceive instances of dancing as making a unique contribution to the life of religion, and to perceive instances of religion as enabled in their meaning by the act of dancing. These concepts and those derived from them in Chapters 8 and 9 suggest questions a scholar can ask, the elements of the culture she can notice. They guide her to examine processes of physical training, education, and social development; enabling environments, architectural spaces, and communal organizations; and the economic, political, and familial dynamics that sustain the action. They focus attention on how accomplishing certain movements effects the meaning of what is represented by making and enacting a logic of a body becoming in and through a spiraling movement of culture. In short, such concepts represent the constructions of a Western scholar who is actively courting the appearance of phenomena that engage and resist the hegemony of verbal forms over Western understandings of religion.

In the end, van der Leeuw's phenomenological analysis of religion and dance belies the simplicity of his initial affirmation: dance can appear as a holy act *but* dance and religion never *unite* in fact or truth, in theory or method. To assume that a dance can meet some criteria and be religious, or to assume that some religious phenomena meets some criteria as dance is to assume that dance and religion are two different entities whose relationship is external to what it means for each phenomenon to be dance or religion. To assume unity is to prevent it. There is no such thing as "religious" art in contrast with "profane" art; or aesthetic religion in contrast to non-aesthetic religion. In van der Leeuw's words, religion and art meet only at the horizon of human possibility: "In silence, religion and art meet and interpenetrate. Religion and art are parallel lines which intersect only at infinity" (S 333; W 460). In the end, the "unity" of dance and religion remains a fruit of phenomenological practice—a fruit of taking dance seriously as kinetic images illuminating the common participation of religion and art in the logic of bodily becoming and the cultural spiral of discovery and response.

Nevertheless, while the "complete unity" of dance and religion is neither conceivable nor desirable, this *consciousness* of religion and dance as parallel lines that "meet and interpenetrate" in the silence of an image-maker's devotion to experience *is* both conceivable and desirable. As suggested above, consciousness of this difference is what will enable continued apprehension of their coincidence. Moreover, the difference between religion and dance serves to sustain the health of both dance and religion as independent checks on one another. As van der Leeuw concludes: "Art is not a province of life . . . Art participates in all of life, and all of life participates in it. Just as the whole of life, it has its origin elsewhere . . . Therefore we need again and again the independence of art as a defense against the imperialism of scientific or dogmatic thought" (S 332; W 461). For scholars, "art" sustains the freedom from "theology" in the form of either transcendent method or truth for which scholars working in and out of the emergence narrative desire. Art does so in so far as it represents a creative act—a disciplined exercise of a particular set of human sensibilities. It can provide a critical perspective on the theories, methods, and conclusions of religious studies by providing a context within which to appreciate the practice of scholarship itself as a full-bodied *art of understanding*.

REVIVING VAN DER LEEUW

I doubt whether anyone else reading the work of van der Leeuw would come up with the reading I have in these pages. What appears in this book is not van der Leeuw per se, but my recreation of the experience that reading his recreated experiences catalyzed in me. My reading and recreation are mediated by my experiences studying philosophy and theology in modern, postmodern, and feminist forms, and by my experiences studying and practicing modern dance. What appears to me in his work, then, is a path towards affirming a generative tension between these two activities and my commitments to them. Van der Leeuw provides me with resources for a new reading of religious studies—one featuring theories and methods amenable to considering dance as both object and resource for scholarship.

Moreover, in reading van der Leeuw this way, my intent is not to rediscover him as some kind of postmodern thinker. He is not. He was one of what Michel Foucault called the "great writers," or the "universal intellectuals," seeking to encompass wholes of meaning within which myriad disparate elements of human experience appear in their significance.[1] He did not believe that any human phenomenon was any more out of his range of impossible/possible understanding than his actions of yesterday; and he articulated an orientation towards scholarship that reflected those beliefs. The contexts within which he sought the meaning of phenomena were not delimited geographically or temporally, but rather, conceptually, experientially, and theologically. He performed the majority of his research on cultures other than his own within the walls of his study, seated in a chair, poring over books. He conducted his studies as a Christian. He used terms that have fallen out of favor for the ways in which they colonize, homogenize, and repress differences—in particular, those distinguishing cultures, genders, races, and classes. Even so, my reading of his writing is informed by sympathies I share with postmodern and feminist scholars who voice such criticisms, such that I am able to discern ways in which he resists these criticisms of his work and offers resources for contemporary thinkers interested in furthering the debates on how to encourage change without repeating the "sins of the fathers." Two points may be made here in van der Leeuw's favor.

First, van der Leeuw makes no pretensions to do otherwise than engage in acts that totalize and subjugate. With refreshing honesty he admits that what he is doing is to cast a net over the variety of the given, a net whose every toss conspires to constitute "reality." For van der Leeuw, the act of attributing or experiencing meaning functions to subjugate that which is thereby "understood." As he insists, "every art and every culture, is an act of [conquest]" (S 289; W 278). Such is the power of representation and its effects.

Yet van der Leeuw is not fatalistic. He believes that there are ways to wield the power of representation responsibly, for embedded in the same totalizing rhythms that enable conquest lie possibilities for understanding and for love. This, for van der Leeuw, is what his "indirect" phenomenological method is about: practicing understanding as love. By cultivating empathy, through the conscious exercise of imagination, a person approaches a human artifact or event as closely as possible, and allows the difference of that "other" to affect her and the appearance of its meaning to her. As van der Leeuw's phenomenologist rehearses the vital, sustaining rhythm of understanding, it becomes what van der Leeuw claims it is, namely the source and center of one's "being in the world" (OU 410). As he writes, "all understanding rests upon self-surrendering love. Were that not the case, then not only all discussion of what appears in religion, but all discussion of appearance in general, would be quite impossible; since to him who does not love, nothing whatever is manifested" (REM 684). Without an open, respectful, willingness to surrender her self to appearances of meaning, a scholar will remain oblivious to the complex tensions and paradoxes characteristic of religion; nothing will appear. In this way, in his phenomenological method, van der Leeuw devises a practice for inciting an "insurrection of subjugated knowledges," and resisting a word-based, science-bound hegemony that continues to reign over postmodern imaginations.[2]

In these respects, van der Leeuw demonstrates a methodological candor rare among philosophers and theologians of the modern West.

He is willing and able to articulate the personal beliefs and commitments that undergird and impel his thinking and writing in the heat of an argument. He is aware of how his theological commitments permeate his phenomenological reflections, not as doctrines to be applied, but as material out of which he re/creates understanding and meaning. He does not pretend to list the coordinates of his social location, as if such a listing would explain or explain away his biases. Rather, he enacts, in his analyses, the eruptions of his thoughts through a mesh of theological images and stories, philosophical concepts, and historical cases. He defiantly holds together the practice of these three disciplines as necessary to a conscious practice of each. I find his ability to jump among discourses, tracing and revealing their interdependencies, inspiring in my attempts to expose how scholars in the field of religion perpetuate, knowingly or unknowingly, a disregard for dance.

In the final analysis, what distinguishes van der Leeuw's writing is his brilliant rendering of the complex relationality between "dance" and "religion" as both studied and practiced in the modern West. His historical and phenomenological research discloses a palpably present absence of dance—an absence he helps us read as a potential for rebirth.

CHAPTER 10

Dancing Religion

> It does not pay to strive for it, for we do not attain it. It is granted us as a rare, disconcerting miracle.
>
> —Gerardus van der Leeuw, *Sacred and Profane Beauty: The Holy in Art*

So far my discussion of van der Leeuw has followed a traditional paradigm: a scholar devises a method which enables him to make sense of a given set of phenomena by guiding his reflections on those phenomena in ways which generate knowledge. Yet, as is hinted at the beginning of Chapter 7, the reverse of this narration may be true as well: namely, that van der Leeuw's interest in dance as religion—however sparked initially—may have impelled and informed his efforts to define religion and devise an indirect method capable of encompassing attention to dance as religion. The imprint of his image of dance on his description of his phenomenology of religion is evident. As noted, a phenomenologist moves incessantly, back and forth across the terrain of human history and the boundaries of her own understanding. A phenomenologist is a mediating thread, roving among social scientific, historical, and theological studies. She participates in the paradox of expression enacted by dance; she makes the movements of culture which dance discloses. In this reverse trajectory, then, images of dance appear as a resource or muse for those developing theories and methods in the study of religion.

Following this trajectory a step further, this chapter considers the implications for the field of thinking about religion and the study of it as a species of dancing. What will scholars see, what questions will they ask, what approaches will they engage if they conceive of religion as a kind of dance—as rhythmic bodily movement enacting a logic of bodily becoming and a cultural spiral of discovery and response? What new perspectives on the field open if scholars take dancing alongside writing as a paradigm for defining the objects, methods, and goals of studying religion?

In this final chapter, then, I reverse the flow of this book to show how theories and methods developed to accommodate dance may help scholars in the field to move beyond the fixation with theology that narrows their responsiveness to media other than words. In the light of this argument, the importance of attending to dance as object and resource for religious studies appears, as does the ongoing relevance of van der Leeuw's work.

AT THE MARGIN

As the first four chapters of this book explain, it is not by accident that dance assumes a marginal position within the study of religion, within the academy at large, and within the culture of the modern West. The place of dance at the margin is a function of the approach to knowledge that sustains these institutions—that is, the assumptions about what counts as knowledge and how to gather it. The basic belief that detachment from the contents of sensory experience plus reflection upon the contents and conditions of those experiences equals objective knowledge, accurate and verifiable, is a powerful paradigm that I cannot help invoking even as I sit and write about dance. My sense that I am doing something and not nothing—even if my intent is to trace the limits of words—depends upon my conviction that *by writing* I can separate my reflections from my lived existence and communicate something that may make sense to someone else. I believe in the act of writing. Writing is the practice that enables me to make a mark in Kant's public realm—a mark that is, and is not, mine. In writing, I rehearse my ability to free my reason. Even as I acknowledge its conditioning, I experience writing's power and find proof of the belief that sustains my efforts.

Within this paradigm, "religion" appears as the name for a problem and dance, a casualty of trying to solve it. Religion names a phenomenon that appears as laying claim to knowledge that cannot be authorized by reason reflecting on experience—that is, through the practice of writing. The implication is that any attempt to study religion participates in a paradox that both enables study and renders it impossible. To study religion is to admit both that someone somewhere is making a claim that appears to exceed the reach of reason, and that translating that claim into rational form is a worthwhile activity.[1] To try to make sense of (what appears as) religion, whether that sense is understood as a process of explanation, interpretation, or understanding, represents an effort to deliver the phenomenon that appears as religion into terms other than its own, terms within which it may be appreciated, respected, demystified—in short, brought into relation with the scholars who seek to study it. The medium for this translation is writing: and dancing, where it appears, reveals its value or contribution to scholarly understandings of religion in so far as it yields to verbal forms. As Kierkegaard's Silentio suggests, it is this faith in writing that enables us to notice dancing as religion while preventing us from understanding it on its own terms.

Given this paradigm, any attempt to acknowledge dance as making a distinctive contribution to religion that cannot be translated challenges the epistemological belief in writing that undergirds the field—the belief that humans can acquire what is important to know about religion through methods of analysis that exercise the freedom, even in limited doses, of reason over and against experience. To take dance seriously as religion is not just to add another object to the pantheon of religious phenomena; it is to call into question the model of knowing within which the study of religion arises as a problem that can be solved in the first place. The location of dance at the margin is intrinsic to how knowledge has been conceived and pursued in Western culture.

Within the field of religious studies, moreover, attention to dance exacerbates the already everpresent sense of vulnerability among scholars of religion concerning the scientific merits of their field. To claim that religion exists is already dubious to many outside of the field in the academy for the reasons just noted. If "religion" can be translated into rational terms, then how is the study of "it" any different from the study of the history, literature, or anthropology that comprise it? Conversely, if religion calls our attention to a unique entity in the world, one that resists rational explanation, then how is the objective study of it possible? For some, any claim to an irreducibility suggests a hidden bias—an unsubstantiated leap of faith in the possibility that something like the sacred exists. This vulnerability finds expression in scholars' hostility towards theology and this hostility drives allegiance to writing as a mode and model of scholarship. Thus, to suggest that religion is a kind of dance appears to heighten this vulnerability by associating religion with a phenomenon that resists translation into the tools and terms of scholarship. Attention to dance exacerbates the vulnerability of the field in so far as its relation to writing appears to parallel the relation of writing to "the sacred."

Enlightenment paradigms of knowledge, while prevalent, are nonetheless under attack from a wide array of sources—feminist, postmodern, postcolonial, and critical theorists. These critiques converge on several themes: reason is embodied; reason is implicated in relations of power; reason is enabled by historical context and tradition; experience is conditioned.[2] Given the cast of these critiques, the time is ripe for attending to the kind of challenge and resource dance provides. Dance names an embodied phenomenon whose meaning cannot be fully translated into verbal forms—a phenomenon known through attention to traces left in kinetic and visual memory; a phenomenon that appears as a crossing of horizontal and vertical planes. Yet, in the case of dance, what appears to elude the reach of rational writing is not an Other realm or being, but rather the transformation of bodily experience that dancing effects. As a result, attempts to develop theories and methods of religion capable of accommodating dance as making a distinct contribution to the field may serve to help scholars respond to critiques of Enlightenment paradigms of knowledge. Attention to dance may help scholars negotiate the moments of affirmation and critique implied by the term "religion" in ways that do not seek justification in a hostility towards theology.

In brief, where scholars approach religion as a species of dance, they may come to reconceive the relationship between reason and experience embraced by seminal thinkers in the field as a generative paradox of expression. Recall that for van der Leeuw, a paradox of expression refers to a contested, vibrant relationship between image and movement animated in every act of communication. This "movement" invokes experience—Schleiermacher's fleeting moment of intuiting and feeling the universe; Hegel's driving moment of negation; Kierkegaard's leap of faith. "Image," by contrast, invokes the privilege of reason over experience—Kant, Descartes, and Silentio's freedom to *see* from a comfortable distance, to reflect upon experience and arrest its truth. As observed in Chapters 1 through 4, the study of religion emerges in the pendulum swing arcing back and forth between positions privileging a kind of reason and those privileging a kind of experience. At stake in what prevails is whether the study of religion affirms or undermines the practice of religion, that is, whether scholars succumb to the temptation of "theology" either by hewing too closely to tradition or by placing too much stock in a transcendent method over and against the particulars of religious life.

By contrast, for dance to appear as itself religion, an expression of power, it must be true at once that sensory experience is informed and enabled by rational reflection (the movement is ordered) and that rational reflection is informed and enabled by bodily being (or else the movement adds nothing to mental life). Both of these dynamics must be true if dance is to appear as something more than a mere body in motion, or a text whose forms are given by intellectual paradigms or whose meaning is inscribed by culture or religion. Both dynamics must hold to consider dance as participating actively in the logic of bodily becoming and the culture spiral of discovery and response. Thus, when dance as dance appears to someone as religion, it does so by revealing religion as encompassing a defiantly dialectical relation between reason and experience—a dynamic, bi-directional, generative connection whose movement produces meaning of different kinds, both conceptual and kinesthetic. As argued in the following pages, this insight is rich with implications for the study of religion. Where religion as a phenomenon is conceived along the lines of dance, rather than along the lines of written texts, then the kinds of phenomena a scholar seeks, the kinds of questions she asks, her very sense of what she is doing in studying religion, all shift. Below I consider some of these implications for attending to the bodily dimensions of religious life; for defining religion; for reconceiving the relation of scholars to phenomena that appear to them; and for mapping future agendas for the field of religious studies.

FROM BODY TO EMBODIMENT

Where religion appears as dance, religion is beautiful movement, requiring nothing other than a human body. This association opens van der Leeuw's complex network of terms as a resource for addressing the fascination with "the body" that pervades the study of religion and the academy at large.[3] Though van der Leeuw's terms are schematic, their range suggests ways to draw together various discourses on the body. In particular, his terms address a rift that has appeared in the body literature between the sociological approaches (in which bodies appear as the site where social meanings are inscribed) and psychological or psychoanalytic approaches (where the body describes the site where unconscious desires are played out).[4] For both approaches, even where they highlight bodily practice, the body is an object that is made to matter by processes external to consciousness. The body in effect disappears in the matrices of relationships that determine its meaning.

The above discussion of van der Leeuw can help identify the agency implied by bodily being and thus highlight the contributions rhythmic bodily movement makes to the study and practice of religion. By approaching religion through the lens of dance, the kinds of questions scholars can ask about the body shift. Instead of asking what do people do with bodies (as if the body is a fixed entity, animated at will), they may ask, what do human bodies become by performing a given set of movements? Instead of asking what is the meaning of bodily acts (as if meaning existed as a detachable statement), they may ask, what are the possibilities for meaning and experience being discovered and recreated by the patterns of (in)attention required to make the movements of religion? Instead of asking what is a person feeling and experiencing in religion (as if a body exists independent of religion), they may ask, how is a person's performing of religion bringing into being as real his relation to the tradition he cites, to the members of his community, to his own past, present, and future self?

Where dance takes precedence as the figure for religion, then religion appears as a process of bodily transformation in which possibilities for meaning and experience are opened and closed by the intention, attention, and effort required to make *ordered movements*. From this perspective, claims to power or efficacy made in the name of religion may be honored as a representation of the transformation wrought through doing. Here, van der Leeuw's interpretive kaleidoscope can guide the investigation to focus on the interplay of the participants' bodily becoming and the community's ongoing evolution.

DYNAMIC DEFINITION

The identification of religion as a form of dance also carries implications for the kinds of definitions adequate to phenomena of religion. In the current scene, as noted earlier, some scholars advocate thin theories close to the ground as guides to noticing the features of phenomena that will help a scholar interpret them as religion. Others advocate thicker theories whose objective methods guarantee accurate and verifiable explanation of religious behavior. Yet for either view, the definition of religion produced by these theories is static— it serves as a framework whose stability acts as a prototype for the kinds of statements about religion that count as adequate translations—however "adequate" is defined. This situation proves awkward in attempts to decide whether or not a given phenomenon is religion. The word "religion" hovers as an arbitrary designation, a scholar's construction, which may or may not fit.

By contrast, where religion is dance, then any definition of religion must be recognized as inherently dynamic. What "religion" is, is always in the process of being determined by a scholar's recreation of the forms in and through which phenomena appear to him as religion. Religion represents an ever-evolving process through which something comes to have meaning for someone as religion. Such a dynamic definition moves across the distinction of insider versus outsider: something may appear as "religion" to either. It suggests that religion is not what a person believes, nor what he has or does per se. Religion rather exists *in the moment of its performances as a kind of doing that embodies a person in relation to a sense of the world*—a sense that may be represented as a relation to a tradition or as a belief in an Other. The relevant question for studying religion becomes: how and why and to what end does some phenomenon have meaning for someone as the terms or conditions of his embodiment? This perspective is especially helpful when confronting the range of folk, popular, cultic, and magical practices that scholars wrestle to include in, or exclude from, their definitions of religion. Where religion is not a system of ideas and practices that a person does or does not engage, but a matrix of performances through which the moments of life appear as meaningful to someone in the form of a tradition or Truth, then it is possible and valuable to ask questions about what kinds of forms come to life through these performances as the condition and context of a person's embodying action.

A TRANSFORMING RELATION

Yet, if religion is a dynamic process of becoming body and generating culture, how is a scholar to secure an objective perspective on religion? Building on the analyses in the chapters above, I argue that the study of religion itself is a transformative process in which both a scholar and the object of her study are transformed, and that in these trans-formations lie both the authority and the responsibility of a scholar.

When religion appears in the form of dance—where the meaning of a phenomenon lies in the experiential knowledge energized in the action of performing—then *the process of coming to understand religion changes the someone who knows*. A person cannot come to an understanding of religion as dance without drawing out webs of his sensory kinetic experience. As he gathers webs of experiential consciousness, he makes that consciousness real, significant as the condition for his understanding. In the action of coming to know, he generates a capacity for deeper insights. The hours spent in devoted attention to the shapes of human experience engage and inform a scholar's own capacity for experiencing appearances. In the action of pursuing understanding, he is moved; the pleasure of understanding enhances, refines, and guides his sensory engagement with the world, as the matrix through which he appears as the one gathering knowledge and insight. More becomes possible. In this way, then, every act of embodied understanding transforms the medium through which further understanding is possible. As such, the push towards objective scholarship mimics a pursuit of an ever-receding horizon: with every step, a scholar strengthens his ability to see and walk farther. Van der Leeuw's appeal for infinite correction, then, is not a function of a belief in a transcendent or objective beyond, but rather an implication of his acknowledgment that understanding is a relationship between an embodied scholar and what can appear to him.

Moreover, in addition to engaging and renewing the subjectivity of the scholar, this pursuit also alters the object of study, namely religion. *The project of studying religion cannot not produce more and different religion in addition to producing new perspectives on religion, regardless of how determined a scholar may be to explain religion away.* To study a culture or tradition is to enter into a relationship with it and (if there are any) its living members. To name elements of a culture or tradition as "religion," in turn, introduces a self-consciousness mediated by a matrix of relationships which includes and extends far beyond the relationship between a scholar and what appears to her as religion. Members of a given tradition invoke these matrices as they appropriate concepts in order to articulate their own sense of their tradition's identity, distinction, and value in relation to other "religions." Whether representatives of that culture embrace that relationship, and use the term "religion" to organize, articulate, and defend the unique character of their "religion," or whether they reject the term, inventing their own terms for how they conceive of their living (such as "lifeway" among Native American Indians), regardless, the "damage" is done. It cannot not be done. The act of breaking open possibilities for communication and understanding is violent, or rather, transforming. As soon as a community or person becomes an object of study for someone, they enter an irreversible process of transformation, entering the community constituted by debate over appearances of meaning.

This dynamic has been particularly true in the case of dance. In so far as theories of religion and methods of studying it have carried built-in biases against dance as religion, scholars have participated in erasing dance from the cultures in which dance appears and has appeared as an integral dimension of the rituals, symbols, texts, and art otherwise recognized as "religion." In most documented cases, the effect of western imperialism has been to eradicate, repress, or marginalize dance occurring in and as religion around the world, whether it is the classical temple dances of India or the tribal dances among Native Americans. The story of how the study of religion has participated in the erasure of dance from human culture is entwined with the histories of missionary activity and colonialism, and more recently with the globalization of culture. It is a story that needs to be told.

In so far as understanding religion changes religion, then, scholars of religion are embroiled in a situation whose ethical implications extend well beyond their particular intentions and actions in relation to the communities they study. *Scholars must take responsibility for their participation in the life of religion.* The challenge they face is to resist as much as possible the limitations on their understanding imposed by the concepts of religion that nonetheless enable them to notice phenomena as worthy of study and capable of translation into rational terms, or at the very least, as capable of being described. The point is not to develop concepts and methods that match actual reality. Theories and practices cannot and never will be thin or transparent enough; nor is there any "thing" there. The point is rather to acknowledge one's own participation in rhythms of submission and mastery, proximity and distance deployed in the act of understanding.

The implication of this situation is not that the fruits of phenomenological analysis are contaminated by subjective bias, but rather that the standards for objectivity dwell as a function of the community for whom "religion" has meaning—the community of scholars and practitioners drawn into being by their shared investment in the term. Objectivity, in other words, is worked out in contests among those with a stake in the phenomenological recreations of religion as they refer to and consult historical examples, contexts, precedents, and theological records. At each turn, the conversation must stretch, twist, and reshape its participants' understandings of religion in ways that enhance the experience of whomever chooses (or is forced) to be involved. As discussed earlier, convergence is not a reasonable goal. What counts as objectivity is a function of an open-ended debate whose value lies in the kind of community created by that debate. Whether or not that community perpetuates hierarchical structures of colonialism, patriarchy, and racism, for example, depends upon the willingness of scholars enabled by these structures to practice vulnerability to appearances of another's meaning and be transformed.

Even so, does this reading not imply that every individual or community produces its own truth about religion such that agreement on topics of religion is rendered impossible? Is the stance or style of life constituting membership in every community simply relative to every other? If so, how is understanding between and among people possible at all? Van der Leeuw offers a response to this nest of questions with his metaphor of the horizontal and vertical planes. The diversity of perspectives on religion represented by scholars claiming to study it may be construed as parallel lines meeting only at the horizon. The lines appear to intersect at the limit of human understanding for those who acknowledge that limit as a critique of particular forms adopted in the present—for those who cultivate an awareness of their phenomenological and historical conditioning. To the extent that a given scholar or religious community employs categories generated in the modern Western study of religion to articulate their identity and difference within the world—regardless of whether they embrace, qualify, reject, or replace those terms—they assume a common *human* horizon. The multiple, overlapping communities of accountability created through various acts of religious study may span a range of different communities and traditions separated by time and place. Such communities have meaning as a forum within which the differences they span may be articulated in debates over the definition of "religion." Here, then, the community of accountability exists in a generative, transformative tension with the worlds represented by scholars and practitioners.

To summarize, conceiving religion on the model of dancing clarifies how and why any attempt to study religion is implicated in the life of religion itself. *Any person attempting to reach the horizon experiences her own displacement as a function of the transforming effort that her reaching exerts on her receptivity to new appearances of meaning.* This dynamic is what van der Leeuw's image of dance as enacting the unity of life makes intelligible. When scholars conceive of religion as dance, it is impossible for them to dismiss the affirmative moment within the scientific project (where the existence of claims that surpass reason is admitted) as a lingering artifact of theological origins. The kind of phenomenon religion is requires participation if it is to be understood. The claim here is not that only an "insider" can really know what is happening in religion, as if religion were a matter of assenting to a shared circle of beliefs. Rather, the claim is that nothing appears as religion to one who is not willing to practice leaping, to affirm that something has meaning for someone, perhaps even because of the way in which it eludes the grasp of writing. As van der Leeuw's attention to dance as religion suggests, it is the inability or unwillingness to acknowledge that vertical expressions of power are implicated in horizontal expressions of power (such as understanding) that breeds authoritarianism, absolutism, immobile images, fixed horizons of possibility, hostility towards theology—and, of course, hostility towards dance.

There is no pure religion. No pure theology. No pure study of religion. Only a messy contested web of interdependent, mutually generative relations. Where an object bears the form of a revelation, a scientific approach to it requires correction by theology. Only when committed to the process of inviting and sustaining such mutual critique can a phenomenologist remain open to ongoing appearances of meaning.

RETURN TO WRITING

Finally, approaching religion as a species of dance carries implications for how scholars conceive of and practice writing. As discussed throughout this book, scholars in religious studies have sought recourse, often unconsciously, to practices of writing in order to authorize a distinction between reason and experience that allows "religion" to emerge as an object of investigation, regardless of whether a given scholar privileges reason or experience, their dialectical reconciliation or irreducible difference. Writing has provided a model and a practice for policing an unstable distinction between religion and the study of it by enacting and exercising the freedom of reason over and against theology in its rational and experiential forms. However, where religion is dance, the ability of writing to perform this task is called into question. Its value for the project of study changes.

Where religion is dance, the value of writing appears in the way the intention to write and the act of writing enable a relationship between scholars and what appears to them as religion. In the act of writing, scholars engage the medium of living in rhythmic, patterned, embodied movement as a process for gathering and mobilizing elements of their experience in the recreation of forms that appear to them—forms they then impose on the world as representing its order. As a bodily practice, writing cultivates a select subset of human capacities as the locus for acquiring, storing, and communicating knowledge. The practice of writing cultivates scholars' vulnerability to appearances of meaning that confirm their experience of writing. If writing is the dominant medium through which they live, then scholars will tend to catch and recreate appearances of meaning that conform to the rhythmic structure and embodied experience they exercise in the action of writing. They will notice what they know how to write down. In the process of writing down what they notice, they will prove to themselves the power of writing in establishing relations of understanding with phenomena, both human and natural, in the world. They will generate themselves as scholars, becoming the "I" that thinks through verbal language as a medium of making religion real and intelligible. They may also succumb to the dangers of representation van der Leeuw describes and convince themselves that they are delivering a "last word." Where scholars practice writing as a medium of stabilizing scholarly detachment, they run the risk of locking themselves into a self-defeating antithesis against "theology" as a cipher for that which threatens the authority of writing and its transparency to truth.

In meeting this challenge, in developing consciousness of writing as embodied activity, scholars may again turn to dance as a resource. Here, as described in the Conclusion to Part 2, dance is helpful in so far as it represents a *practice* that exercises attention along the vector described here as moving from experience to reason. Dancing may employ and thus strengthen scholars' range of awareness concerning the dynamism of their own bodily becoming. Dancing in this sense does not afford access to some primal experience or to the body per se. Rather it raises *physical consciousness* by enacting the process by which people discover and respond to the world, recreating themselves and the meaning of their environments by recreating the rhythmic, kinetic, and visual forms in which these environments appear to them. Practiced in this way, dancing may open up a perspective on writing as participating in a paradox of expression. It may help to exercise rational thinking in ways that are conducive to understanding bodily dimensions of religious life. It may help scholars become aware of how they are creating *themselves*, seizing and discarding the rhythms of life, as they write.

For van der Leeuw, the performance and practice of dance exercises *knowledge*—not just a technical know-how, but rather, an understanding of self and world within which such practice is valued as significant. As such, dance does not represent a flip side of words; it offers something else—a different perspective from which to read words as images. As van der Leeuw concludes, "the life of the dance has an independent existence. It awakes the serene knowledge of spiritual release, and the blessed consciousness of being transported by a sovereign power. The surrender of oneself to a stronger power, the unification [literally, 'getting in gear'] of one's own movements with the movement of the whole, is what makes dance religious" (S 68; W 90). The possibility of this consciousness is what van der Leeuw's analysis demonstrates on phenomenological grounds.

FUTURE AGENDAS

Since van der Leeuw wrote his second edition of *Wegen en Grenzen* in 1948, some of the aesthetic and cultural developments that he predicted have come to pass. Several forms of dance, most notably ballet and modern dance, have secured recognition as fine arts. These forms have inspired Christians to make dances for inclusion in worship services, and representatives of many other religious traditions—Native American, Japanese, Tibetan Buddhist, African, Caribbean, Classical Indian, Hispanic, and others—to develop their dances into proscenium forms for Western audiences. There remains much work to be done to understand, guide, and nourish these developments.

Here, van der Leeuw's braided approach provides a helpful map for bridging developments in the study and practice of dance with those in the study and practice of religious studies. Contributions by a diverse group of scholars and religious representatives are necessary—a group whose contested unity will appear by virtue of each member's decision to participate in the process of naming structural relations binding appearances of dance and of religion. First, more historical and social scientific accounts of dance in world history are needed by anthropologists, ethnologists, archeologists, sociologists, and historians of various kinds to help stir up the scant evidence that remains from times and places where "dance" occurred. Such evidence is difficult to gather and assess given the ephemeraland lived character of dance as movement. Historical methods for interpreting images of dance and accounts of dance are needed as well, as are projects that revisit the material already metabolized into the western world. References to dance have been overlooked. Dance is mute and has been muted. As such, careful attention to its silencing is important, especially in text-based traditions with strong historical voices.

In addition, "theologians" or representatives speaking from and for various traditions are also needed to reflect on the meaning of dance from their perspectives, in the context of their symbolic universes, especially when forms from their histories are being westernized for the stage. Such theological reflections provide historians with material and guidance, even as they mine the work of historians in identifying salient moments of their histories. More importantly, however, such reflections begin to correct the absence of dance from religious self-representations informed by the terms generated by Western scholars of religion, ignorant as they have been of dance. Representatives of various traditions can revisit the ways in which their appropriation of phenomenological categories has shaped their understanding of their own dance forms and question the influence of those terms.

Within Christian circles, some progress has been made on this front. However, most writers on Christianity and dance are limited by their phenomenological understanding of dance. Their apologies for dance treat dance as a "thing" existing *outside* of Christian religion that must be drawn into the Christian circle.[5] They ignore the fact that they appeal to an image of dance which is indebted to early modern dancers, that the aesthetic forms of modern dance were always already steeped in religious imagery, language, and commitments, and that even their images of Christianity as justifying the inclusion of "dance" are informed by experiences of modern dance. To the extent that such writers consider "dance" and "Christian religion" as two entities, they miss the structural relations between the two that van der Leeuw seizes upon as a promise for a renewed consciousness of dance as an expression of life.

In addition then to historical, social scientific, humanist, and theological voices, a third kind of project is necessary, one akin to van der Leeuw's phenomenological method. As a phenomenologist, van der Leeuw respects the *historicity* of both "dance" and "religion" as structures, and acknowledges that it is impossible to wield these terms independent of the net of embodied particulars which each represents. He does not assume an easy reconciliation, as if "dance" might be subsumed within religious practice as a medium of expression transparent to words. Nor does van der Leeuw mute the critical potential of dance vis-à-vis theory and method in the study of religion. He owns the historicity of his own phenomenological categories, their dependence upon emergent cultural forms, and their support in the theological images of God's incarnating movement, reflected and reenacted in human love, which have meaning for him. He gestures towards a future on the basis of a present which answers to promises residing in his perceptions of the past. He invokes a "maternal rhythm" of life in order to affirm and critique particular historical forms leveling claims to ultimacy. Van der Leeuw's phenomenological method opens paths to historical cases beyond his reach whose difference from the cases in his experience serves to enrich phenomenological understanding, historical knowledge, and theological evaluations of "dance." He invites readers to do likewise.

The work has already begun. As the field of religion and dance continues to grow, van der Leeuwian phenomenological studies of historical accounts and theological reports will be crucial to the process of developing terms of analysis capable of drawing historical and theological perspectives on dance into a healthy, generative contestation at the point of their common appeal to "religion." Dance has evolved new forms of expression, and so too must historical and theological accounts concerning what it is about dance as art that renders it capable of appearing as a conduit for experiences of power.

Notes

Preface

1. Nietzsche, Friedrich. *The Portable Nietzsche* (1954), 406.
2. Graham, Martha. *Blood Memory* (1991), 5.
3. Margaret Miles is another scholar of religion who makes this observation and assesses the implications for theory and method in the study of religion. She focuses on visual images in paintings and architecture, arguing that language users need practice in critical image use in order to understand the experiences of non-language users. See *Image as Insight* (1985) and *Carnal Knowing* (1991).
4. For an excellent summary of this quandary, see Susan Foster, *Reading Dancing* (1986), xiv-xv.
5. This discussion echoes the contrast Talal Asad makes between symbolic representation and disciplinary practice in his *Genealogies of Religion* (1993). His point is that the fields of anthropology and religious studies are predicated on the assumption that bodily action is symbolic representation and therefore capable of being interpreted, translated. He contrasts that perception with the view of medieval Christians for whom bodily action was a transformative practice—one that opened up capacities for experience and expression that would not otherwise exist.

Introduction

1. Miriam, David, and Judith all dance in celebration of God's gracious actions on their behalf (Exod. 15:20; 2 Sam. 6:14-16, 20-23 and 1 Chron. 15:16, 25-29; Judith 15:12-3); the Psalms admonish believers to "Praise him with timbrel and dance" (Ps. 150:4, also Ps. 149:3) and thank God for having "turned for me my mourning into dancing" (Ps. 30:11); the author of Ecclesiastes affirms that "For everything there is

a season, and a time for every matter under heaven . . . a time to
mourn, and a time to dance" (Eccles. 3:1, 4). In the New Testament, the
dance performed by the daughter of Herodias seduces Herod into
granting her mother's wish for the head of John the Baptist (Matt.
14:6; Mark 6:22); Jesus, in describing the "men of this generation"
compares them to children in the market place calling to one another,
"We piped to you and you did not dance; we wailed, and you did not
weep" (Matt.11:16-19; Luke 7:31-4); the elder son to the prodigal,
returning from the field, hears "music and dancing" (Luke 15:25). For
additional references of dance in the Hebrew Bible and their
etymological derivations, see Mayer Gruber, "Ten Dance-Derived
Expressions in the Hebrew Bible," in *Dance as Religious Studies* (Adams
and Apostolos-Cappadona, eds., 1990). For the cultural and religious
contexts for the biblical references to dance, see W.O.E. Oesterly, *The
Sacred Dance: A Study in Comparative Folklore* (1923). All biblical
quotations are from the Oxford publication of the Revised Standard
Version (1977).

For generous and conservative arguments concerning the presence
of dance in Christian history, see Louis Backman, *Religious Dances in
the Christian Church and in Popular Medicine* (1952), and J.G. Davies,
Liturgical Dance: An Historical, Theological, and Practical Handbook
(1984), respectively.
2. See Sydney Ahlstrom, *A Religious History of the American People*
(1972); Edward Andrews, *The People Called Shakers* (1953); Al
Raboteau, *Slave Religion* (1978); Sterling Stuckey, "Christian
Conversion and the Challenge of Dance," in *Choreographing History*,
edited by Susan Foster (1995).
3. Judith Lynne Hanna, *To Dance Is Human* (1987), Chapter 1.
4. See Deborah Jowitt, *Time and the Dancing Image* (1988), Chapter 1.
5. See Preus (1987) and McCutcheon (1997, 2001) for prominent
examples of this narrative. See Roberts (2004) for a critique.
6. Gerardus van der Leeuw, *Sacred and Profane Beauty: The Holy in Art*
(1963), 271. Hereafter "S." The English version is translated from a
German translation of a Dutch edition that was edited and published
after van der Leeuw's death. See *Wegen en Grenzen. Studie over de
verhouding van religie en kunst* (1948, 1955).
7. See Robert Cummings Neville, "Religious Studies and Theological
Studies," *Journal of the American Academy of Religion* (61:2), 185-200.
8. Michel Foucault, *Power/Knowledge* (1980), 81-2.
9. Asad (1993), Chapter 2.
10. Bell (1997), 81.
11. Foster (1986), and in her essay, "Choreographing History" (1995).
12. Schechner, in Schechner and Appel (1990), 36.

13. For further discussion of these issues, see LaMothe, "Why Dance? Towards a Theory of Religion as Practice and Performance."
14. Catherine Bell, "Modernism and Postmodernism in the Study of Religion," *Religious Studies Review* (1996), 187.
15. It is possible to make the argument that these tools themselves are always already "theological" and cannot *not* be in a religious culture that privileges the Word as the manifestation of God in the world. I agree. The questions that follow include: how do you define "theology" and how do you act when escape from "theology" is impossible? I address these issues in my discussion of van der Leeuw in Part 2.
16. See Clifford Geertz, *Works and Lives: The Anthropologist as Author* (1988), for a discussion of how this dynamic plays out in anthropology.
17. For biographical information, see Ann Daly, *Done into Dance* (1995), and Suzanne Shelton, *Divine Dancer: A Biography of Ruth St. Denis* (1981). For analysis of their cultural contexts and impact, see also Elizabeth Kendall, *Where She Danced: The Birth of American Art-Dance* (1979); Deborah Jowitt, *Time and the Dancing Image* (1988); Ramsey Burt, *Alien Bodies: Representations of Modernity, 'Race' and Nation in Early American Modern Dance* (1998), and Mark Franko, *Dancing Modernism/Performing Politics* (1995).
18. See Kimerer L. LaMothe, "Passionate Madonna: The Christian Turn of Ruth St. Denis," *Journal of the American Academy of Religion* (66:4), 747-769.
19. S 70-1. In the plates that accompany the Dutch editions of this book, van der Leeuw includes a drawing of Isadora Duncan. For an account of her influence on his work, see LaMothe, "Why Dance?"
20. Van der Leeuw published an earlier short work on dance in Dutch and then German which has not been translated into English: *In den hemel is enen dance* (1930); *'In dem Himmel ist ein Tanz 'Uber dies religiose Bedeutung des Tanzes und des Festzuges* (1931). Ideas developed there appear in the first part of *Sacred and Profane Beauty*, in "Beautiful Movement," the section devoted to a discussion of dance. See Chapters 7, 8 and 9 for a discussion of this work.
21. Oesterley (1923). Oesterley's intent in this book was to demonstrate an evolution of liturgical forms from the dance-based, pre-Judaic religions, through the formalized Jewish dance practices, to the internalized worship of the Christian communion. In this schema, dance represents a mode of religious experience and expression depicted as less civilized than Christian forms.
22. See for example, R.R. Marrett, *Faith, Hope and Charity in Primitive Religion* (1932).
23. Sachs argues for a cross-cultural definition of dance as an activity integral to the religious and artistic dimensions of human life, and

attests that dance is on the edge of a renaissance as represented by the emergence of modern dance.

24. Joann Kealiinohomoku, "Dance Ethnology: Where Do We Go from Here?" *Dancing in the Millennium Conference* (July 20, 2000).

25. Johan Huizinga, *Homo Ludens* (1938).

26. Fisk, the daughter and wife of Presbyterian ministers, was one of the first pioneers in choreographing dances for Christian worship services. She called her dancers a "rhythmic choir" in order to avoid the negative connotations of "dance." Margaret Palmer Fisk, *The Art of the Rhythmic Choir* (1950). This book was edited and reissued in 1967 as *A Time to Dance*, under the name of her second husband, Margaret Fisk Taylor.

27. Backman (1952).

28. For a history of the Sacred Dance Guild see: Fisk (1950); Carlynn Reed, *And We Have Danced: A History of the Sacred Dance Guild, 1958-1978* (1978); Toni Intravaia, *And We Have Danced*, Vol. 2 (1994). Today the SDG sponsors yearly conferences and regional workshops, and publishes a journal for its 500-plus members, who span a vast geographical and religious terrain. See *SDG Journal* (1995).

29. Paul Tillich, *Systematic Theology: Volume Three* (1959), 200.

30. Doug Adams founded The Sharing Company as a publisher and clearinghouse for books and articles by members and affiliates of the Sacred Dance Guild. A number of these pamphlets were published together in *Dance as Religious Studies*, edited by Doug Adams and Diane Apostolos-Cappadona (1990). A brief review of the Bibliography supports this description of literature in the field to date. See also Ronald Gagne et al., *Introducing Dance in Christian Worship* (1999).

31. See Judith Rock and Norman Mealy, *Performer as Priest and Prophet: Restoring the Intuitive in Worship through Music and Dance* (1988). Also, Judith Rock, *Theology in the Shape of Dance* (1978); J.G. Davies, "Towards a Theology of the Dance," in his edited volume, *Worship and Dance* (1975).

32. A number of factors contribute to this situation. Often scholars in dance studies draw upon cultural studies for methodological resources, and from this perspective conceive of religion as "ideology." The sense that Christianity is responsible for the marginal status of dance practice and scholarship in the West also hinders attention to questions of religion. Finally, dance scholars share with scholars in religious studies a sense of the acute struggle that is required to secure recognition as a scholarly discipline within an academy that privileges scientific and linguistic paradigms. For this reason alone, I am convinced, the disciplines have much to share with and learn from each other.

For excellent work in dance studies, see especially works in dance theory by Ann Cooper-Albright, Sallie Banes, Ramsey Burt, Susan Foster, Mark Franko, Deborah Jowitt, Susan Manning; in philosophical approaches to dance by Sondra Horton Fraleigh, Maxine Sheets-Johnston, Francis Sparshott; in dance ethnology by Judith Lynne Hanna, Joann Kealiinohomoku, Sallie Ness, Cynthia Novack, Deirdre Sklar; as well as dance anthologies by Ann Dils and Ann Cooper-Albright, Alexandra Carter, Jane Desmond, Roger Copeland and Marshal Cohen, and Sondra Horton Fraleigh.

33. Positions represented, respectively, by Donald Wiebe, "Phenomenology of Religion as Religion-Cultural Quest: Gerardus van der Leeuw and the Subversion of the Scientific Study of Religion," in *Religionswissenschaft und Kulturkritik: Beitrage zur Konfrenz—The History of Religions and Critique of Culture in the Days of Gerardus van der Leeeuw (1890-1950)* (Kippenberg and Luchesi, eds., 1991), 65-86; Thomas Ryba, *The Essence of Phenomenology and Its Meaning for the Scientific Study of Religions* (1991); and Hans Penner, *Impasse and Resolution: A Critique of the Study of Religion* (1989). See also Donald Wiebe, *The Politics of Religious Studies* (1999). See critique of Penner begun by Ursala King in her "Review Essay: Impasse and Resolution," *Journal of the American Academy of Religion* (61/4), 785-92.

PART 1: WRITING AGAINST THEOLOGY

Introduction to Part One

1. For a history of changing definitions of the term "religion" up to the cusp of the modern era, see W.C. Smith, *The Meaning and End of Religion* (1991), and J.Z. Smith, "Religion, Religions, Religious" in Taylor (1998).

1: The Rift in Religion: René Descartes and Immanuel Kant

1. A useful history of European Enlightenment movements, and there were many, remains Peter Gay's. See in particular *The Enlightenment: An Interpretation, Volume II: The Science of Freedom* (1969). Also influential for this chapter is Foucault's reading of Kant in *The Order of Things*. As he writes, "I should like to know whether the subjects responsible for scientific discourse are not determined in their situation, their function, their perceptive capacity, and their practical possibilities by conditions that dominate and even overwhelm them" (xiv). He calls these conditions the "positive unconscious of knowledge" or "rules of formation" that allow a particular order of things to emerge (xi). Foucault identifies the Kantian critique as

marking the threshold of modernity in which questions arise
concerning the limits and enabling conditions of representation.

2. See Stephen Toulmin, "Descartes in His Time," in Descartes, *Discourse on Method and Meditations on First Philosophy* (1996), 121-146.

3. Francis Bacon, *Works 1622-3*, vol. II, 14-5.

4. Ibid.

5. Immanuel Kant, *Critique of Pure Reason* (1965 [1787]), 20 (B xiii). Hereafter, "CPR."

6. For discussion of whether Descartes offers a "metaphysics" in the form of "onto-theo-logy," see Jean Luc Marion, *On Descartes' Metaphysical Prism: The Constitution and the Limits of Onto-theo-logy in Cartesian Thought* (1999). Marion argues that Descartes' formulations of "soul," "God," and the relationship between them represent a "transition" to "the principle of reason" (5), a "metaphysics" redefined in contrast to the ideas of "theology" or "ontology" of his day (66).

7. René Descartes, *Discourse on Method* (1956 [1637]), 11. Hereafter, "DM." See also, René Descartes, "Meditations II and III," in *Discourse on Method and Meditations on First Philosophy* (1996). Hereafter, "M."

8. See also Descartes, M, 100.

9. For a discussion and critique of the physiological basis of Descartes' imaginative act, see Drew Leder, *The Absent Body* (1990).

10. DM, 24. See also M, Sixth Meditation, 96-108.

11. There are many ways to critique Descartes' insistence on this distinction between reason and experience, as subsequent theorists demonstrate. My point here is to note how it functions to enable his ideas of God and religion.

12. This possibility of elevating the idea of God to critique the forms of religion is foreshadowed in his method itself. As he describes, while rejecting all beliefs, Descartes finds it prudent to maintain a "provisional code of morality," subject to whatever standards of evaluation he eventually locates as true (DM 15).

13. For evidence of the continuing relevance of this essay, see Talal Asad, *Genealogies of Religion*, Chapter 6, "Religious Criticism in the Middle East." While Asad affirms that Kant can not be considered a "representative" of the Enlightenment "as a whole," he holds that "Kant's text may nevertheless be taken as marking a formative moment in the theorization of a central feature of 'civil society,' the feature concerning the possibilities of open rational criticism" (201-2). See also readings by Habermas (1989) and Foucault (1984).

14. Immanuel Kant, "An Answer to the Question: 'What is Enlightenment?'" *Kant's Political Writings* (1991 [1784]), 54. Hereafter, "WE."

15. Immanuel Kant, "What Is Orientation in Thinking?" *Kant's Political Writings* (1991 [1786]), 240. Hereafter, "WO."

16. Kant elaborates this concept of purposiveness in this third critique, the *Critique of Judgment* (1987 [1793]). Although this *critique* defines art and evaluates various forms of art, dance appears only briefly and then as a mixed art, ranked in value below poetry and music. For a discussion of Kant's aesthetics see Mary McCloskey's *Kant's Aesthetics* (1997).

17. See also Immanuel Kant, *Critique of Practical Reason* (1985 [1788]).

18. WO 243; Immanuel Kant, *Religion within the Limits of Reason Alone* (1960 [1793]), 3. Hereafter "RLR."

19. For a contemporary example of a Christian theologian who develops a theological method influenced by Kant's philosophy of religion, see Gordon D. Kaufman, *In Face of Mystery* (1993).

20. For related discussions of why philosophers in the modern West before the twentieth century do not acknowledge dance as a fine art, see Francis Sparshott, *Off the Ground: First Steps to a Philosophical Consideration of the Dance* (1988). Sparshott argues that dance had not yet emerged as enough of an art to merit such attention—a thesis that raises the question of why dance had not. See also articles in *What Is Dance? Readings in Theory and Criticism* (1983), edited by Roger Copeland and Marshal Cohen.

21. Mary Wollstonecraft in *A Vindication of the Rights of Women* (1792), offers an early example of this critique. For Wollstonecraft, the difference in rational capacity that Kant takes as a natural difference between the sexes is a function of unequal access to educational opportunities. When women are denied exercises in reading and writing on the basis of their sex, they are unable to cultivate an ability to imagine themselves free from the contents and conditions of sensory experience. As she writes, "the conduct and manners of women, in fact, evidently prove that their minds are not in a healthy state; for, like the flowers which are planted in too rich a soil, strength and usefulness are sacrificed to beauty; and the flaunting leaves, after having pleased a fastidious eye, fade, disregarded on the stalk, long before the season when they ought to have arrived at maturity. One cause of this barren blooming I attribute to a false system of education" (1). While Wollstonecraft does not challenge the goal of Kant's program, her critique highlights its dependence on writing as a disciplinary practice. Education is not simply about acquiring information; it is about developing the ability to think critically about one's own embodiment. Wollstonecraft's critique thus supports the idea that the forces driving the marginalization of dance in philosophical discourse are not the association of dance with the body

or with the feminine per se. More important is a willingness to be seduced by the illusions of freedom the experience of writing engenders.

2: Recovering Experience: Friedrich Schleiermacher

1. Wayne Proudfoot makes this case in his book *Religious Experience* (1985). See also Grace Jantzen in *Power, Gender and Christian Mysticism* (1995): "[T]he idea of such a mystical core of religion derives in large part from Schleiermacher's attempt to circumvent Kantian strictures on religious knowledge" (338). Jantzen also exposes how the move to privilege a mystical core of religion represents one of the "technologies of patriarchy": it sustains gender inequities.

   For biographical perspectives, see Brian Gerrish, *A Prince of the Church: Schleiermacher and the Beginnings of Modern Theology* (1984), and Ruth D. Richardson, *The Role of Women in the Life and Thoughts of Early Schleiermacher (1768-1806)* (1991).

2. In what follows, when I talk about Schleiermacher as responding to "Kant," I do not mean to imply that Schleiermacher responds only to Kant, or even primarily to Kant. Rather, I am interested in contrasting Schleiermacher's position with the kind of position Kant represents— whether held by a scholar in the nineteenth century or the twenty-first. For a fuller account of the romantic context within which Schleiermacher's response to his cultured despisers arises, see Philippe Lacoue-Labarthe and Jean-Luc Nancy, *The Literary Absolute: The Theory of Literature in German Romanticism* (1988).

3. My analysis of Schleiermacher focuses on his first book because it is here that he develops his use of "religion" as a generic term, and because this text is the one that has proven so influential for subsequent scholars of religion as a position to emulate and/or reject. As professor at the University of Berlin, Schleiermacher went on to complete a landmark work in modern theology, *The Christian Faith* [*Glaubenslehre*], (1989 [1821]).

4. Friedrich Schleiermacher, *On Religion* (1988), 22, my emphasis. Hereafter, "OR."

5. I disagree with Sharf (in Taylor 1998) and others who emphasize that the "experience" Schleiermacher calls "religion" is immediate, subjective, and unexamined. Schleiermacher's point is that the "mysterious moment" of religion represents an inextricable fusion of subject and object prior to any separation of intuition and feeling. As a result, "it" can never fall to one side of an equation. Any characterization of "it" as "immediate" is always already mediated by an act of reason. When read in this way, the proximity of

Schleiermacher and Hegel emerges clearly. See Chapter 3 below. Van
der Leeuw as well will amplify this implication of Schleiermacher's
work in the design of his phenomenological method.

6. For Schleiermacher's description of these feelings see OR 45-6, 51-3.

7. OR 60. Martin Buber develops this distinction into a difference
between an I-Thou "encounter" and an I-It "experience." See Martin
Buber, *I and Thou* (1996), especially "First Part."

8. Schleiermacher's concept of a "mediator" shares much with the
concept of the "poet" developed by his contemporaries in the romantic
movements. For a discussion of Schleiermacher's "theoaesthetics" in
this context, see Mark C. Taylor, *Disfiguring* (1992), Chapter 2.

9. In addition to the effects noted below, this dependence on writing
undercuts Schleiermacher's otherwise positive endorsement of women
as well. Although there is evidence that he wrote other of his texts
with a woman he esteemed and loved and that ideas in *On Religion*
actually derived from letters she had written to him, the authorship of
the text remained his alone. See Richardson (1991) for an exposition of
Schleiermacher's early views on women and their significance for his
arguments in *On Religion*.

10. OR 115. See the "Fifth Speech: On the Religions," 95-124, in general.

3: Doing the Work of Spirit: G. W. F. Hegel

1. The continuing relevance of Hegel's *Phenomenology of Spirit* (1977
[1806], hereafter, "PS") in Hegel's corpus is evident in the wealth of
secondary literature it is currently spawning. See most notably Jean-
Luc Nancy, *Hegel: The Restlessness of the Negative* (2002); Michael N.
Forster, *Hegel's Idea of a Phenomenology of Spirit* (1998); Merold
Westphal, *History and Truth in Hegel's Phenomenology* (1998), and
Terry Pinkard, *Hegel's Phenomenology: The Sociality of Reason*
(1994). See also Robert Pippin, *Hegel's Idealism: The Satisfactions of
Self-Consciousness* (1995).

2. For a comparative discussion of the contents of these lectures, see Peter
Hodgson's "Editorial Introduction" to Hegel's *Lectures on the Philosophy
of Religion: One Volume Edition, The Lectures of 1827* (1988). Hereafter,
"LPR." Hegel may have been initially spurred to give these lectures by
news that "his colleague and rival," Schleiermacher, would be publishing
The Christian Faith (1989 [1821]) (LPR 1). Over the eleven-year period,
his concept of religion remained constant, although his understanding of
the philosophy of religion and his treatment of historical religions
evolved significantly. The difference between the 1827 and 1831 lectures
is largely in the treatment of historical religions (LPR 2-3).

3. PS § 36, 21. In Hegel's words, "experience is the name we give to just
this moment, in which the immediate, the unexperienced, i.e., the

abstract, whether it be of sensuous [but still unsensed] being, or only thought of as simple, becomes alienated from itself and then returns to itself from this alienation, and is only then revealed for the first time in its actuality and truth."

4. In the *Phenomenology of Spirit*, "reason" is not only a human faculty, but also a shape of consciousness that aligns roughly with the European Enlightenment. As a shape of consciousness, Reason (which I will capitalize to distinguish it from the faculty) represents a particular concept and use of human reason. Describing Reason, Hegel writes: "Reason is the certainty of consciousness that it is all reality . . . [the certainty that] 'I am I', in the sense that the 'I' which is an object for me is the sole object, is all reality and all that is present." See PS §233, 140.

5. With this reading, I lay the groundwork for contesting interpretations of Hegel that describe him as a philosopher who elevates "reason" as the highest manifestation of "subjective spirit" (see for example, Charles Taylor, *Hegel* (1975). Such readings of Hegel support the idea that Hegel's community of philosophers excludes women, as argued by Seyla Benhabib in *Situating the Self: Gender, Community and Postmodernism in Contemporary Ethics* (1992), Chapter 8.

6. In a number of places it seems that Hegel denies this capacity of self-consciousness to women as well as to other members of society who are not adult, privileged men. In his discussion of "The ethical order" in the *Phenomenology*, he assigns women to the realm of the family and men to the public realm. For an interpretation and defense of Hegel's argument, see Terry Pinkard, *Hegel's Phenomenology: The Sociality of Reason* (1994). Pinkard defends Hegel's account of the "bourgeois patriarchal family" as "well suited to play an essential role in modern social life" (304), even if it is not palatable by some contemporary standards.

   For a range of critical responses, see *Feminist Interpretations of G.W.F. Hegel* (1996), edited by Patricia Mills. For a political philosophy that finds resources for a "Hegelian feminism" in an alternative reading of Hegel, see Kimberley Hutchings, *Hegel and Feminist Philosophy* (2003), and LaMothe, "Reason, Religion and Sexual Difference" (2005).

7. LPR 121. See also 120, 162, 167-8.

8. For a discussion of Hegel's maternal rhetoric, see Eric Clarke, "Fetal Attraction: Hegel's An-aesthetics of Gender," in *Feminist Interpretations of G.W.F. Hegel* (1996), edited by Patricia J. Mills.

9. As Hegel insists, "The content remains always the same. The true is not for the single spirit but for the world spirit. But for the latter, representation and concept are *one*. The difficult thing is to separate out from a content what pertains only to representation" (LPR 145).

10. While this act of denying one's subjectivity could be construed as hostility to embodiment and embodied others, I would argue that the kind of dismissing Hegel has in mind represents a moment in a dialectical process designed to promote recognition of one's embodied historicity. Though Merold Westphal and others have developed an interpretation of Hegel's *Phenomenology* as a critique of the transcendental subject, more work needs to be done in assessing the implications of this reading for feminist concerns. See Westphal, *History and Truth in Hegel's Phenomenology* (1998).

11. Ludwig Feuerbach develops the critique of religious faith implied by Hegel's identification of philosophy with ethical life. See *The Essence of Christianity* (1957 [1841]), Chapter 26 in particular.

12. For a discussion of community in Hegel's political and social theory, see Frederick Neuhouser, *Foundations of Hegel's Social Theory: Actualizing Freedom* (2000). See also Hutchings (2003), Chapter 6.

13. Jon Stewart, "Hegel and the Myth of Reason," in *The Hegel Myths and Legends* (1996), 306-7.

4: The Poet and the Dancer: Søren Kierkegaard

1. Examples of references to "dance" or to the "leap" of faith appear in *Either/Or* (by Victor Eremita), *The Concept of Anxiety* (by Vigilius Haufniensis), *Philosophical Fragments* and *Concluding Unscientific Postscript* (by Johannes Climacus), and, as I discuss in detail below, *Fear and Trembling* (by Johannes de Silentio).

2. For a comparison of Hegel and Kierkegaard's theories of selfhood that takes account of other works as well, see Mark C. Taylor, *Journeys to Selfhood: Hegel and Kierkegaard* (1980).

3. Søren Kierkegaard, *Fear and Trembling* (Ed. and Tr. by Howard V. Hong and Edna H. Hong, 1983 [1843]), 7. Hereafter "FT."

4. In writing to make unintelligibility intelligible, Kierkegaard foreshadows his popularity among postmodern theorists interested in writing as a critical category for thinking through the history of philosophy. See discussions in: *Kierkegaard in Post/Modernity* (1995), edited by Martin Matustik & Merold Westphal. See also *Altarity* (1987), in which Taylor frames Kierkegaard as answering Derrida's call to "heed the solicitation of an inconceivable Other" (303). Taylor continues: "The space-time of such erring is the writerly spacing-timing of *Fear and Trembling*" (303).

5. This image of a "rouged and powdered" theology raises the vexing question of Kierkegaard's attitudes towards women that seem conflicted at best. Though I do not engage these issues in depth here, I note that in his time, the most celebrated ballet dancers were female. This fact corroborates his claim in *Fear and Trembling* that the order of knighthood "mak[es] no distinction between male and female" (45).

For the beginnings of much needed discussion, see *Feminist Interpretations of Søren Kierkegaard* (1997), edited by Celine Léon & Sylvia Walsh. For a biographical account, see Walter Lowrie's *A Short Life of Kierkegaard* (1970).

6. Kierkegaard would have had plenty of opportunity to see and read about ballet. Unlike the previous thinkers we have considered, Kierkegaard was writing in the heyday of Romantic Ballet (1830-80s). Moreover, under the leadership of August Bournonville (1828-79), the Royal Danish Ballet was one of the most exciting and productive companies to watch. Though home to many of the romantic artists, poets, and philosophers whose visions inspired the plots and characters of the romantic ballet, the German states were slower to develop their own ballet culture. See Jowitt (1988), Chapter 1. See also Sorrell (1981), "Balletomania."

7. For a perspective on the history of romantic ballet, see Jowitt (1988), Chapter 1; Sorrell (1981). See also, *Rethinking the Sylph: New Perspectives on the Romantic Ballet* (1997), edited by Lynn Garafola. Even though ballet was a popular art at the time, it was not considered a fine art. As Jowitt relates: "[T]he leaders of the Romantic movement in literature and painting—the fiercest balletomanes among them—looked down on ballet even as they delighted in it. It was, they understood, an excuse for watching pretty, lightly clad women disporting themselves. Yet everywhere their prose betrays deeper responses" (33). Kierkegaard may have picked up on these "deeper responses."

8. In *Concluding Unscientific Postscript,* Johannes Climacus acknowledges Gotthold Lessing as the first to use the image of a leap to describe faith as a state of existential commitment that cannot be mediated by historical, logical, or normative criteria and still be what it is. See *Concluding Unscientific Postscript to "Philosophical Fragments"* (1992 [1846]), Volume I, 93-106.

9. For a discussion of Kierkegaard's meditations on the impossibility of writing—in doodling as well as in prose— see Taylor, *Alterity*, Chapter 10. For an approach through Kierkegaard's "aesthetic," see Terry Eagleton, *The Ideology of the Aesthetic* (1990), Chapter 7.

10. Hegel's own prose in the "Preface" to his *Phenomenology of Spirit* suggests his awareness of this dynamic. According to him, his Science is a mere notion—an idea awaiting full realization. Realizing this notion requires participation of humans in developing their dialectical capabilities and acknowledging themselves in doing so as the work of spirit becoming self-consciousness. Thus, Hegel casts his Preface as a call to participate in making his Science real. See discussion of what such participation entails in "Reason, Religion, and Sexual Difference" (LaMothe, 2005).

Conclusion to Part 1: Living the Legacy

1. Friedrich Nietzsche urges his readers to practice "thinking" as a "kind of dancing" (*Twilight of Idols* in *Portable Nietzsche*, 512). For discussion, see LaMothe, *Nietzsche's Dancers: Isadora Duncan, Martha Graham, and the Reevaluation of Christian Values* (2005).

5: A Braided Approach to the Study of Religion: Gerardus van der Leeuw

1. These two are: *Religion in Essence and Manifestation* (1986), hereafter, "REM"; and *Sacred and Profane Beauty: The Holy in Art* (1963); hereafter, "S." Jacques Waardenberg has translated three additional lectures by van der Leeuw, published in Waardenburg, *Classical Approaches to the Study of Religion* (1973), 389-431.
2. For biographical information, see Jacques Waardenburg, "Reflections on the Study of Religion, Including an Essay on the Work of Gerardus van der Leeuw," *Religion and Reason* 15 (1978), 187-92.
3. John Carman, "The Theology of a Phenomenologist: An Introduction to the Theology of Gerardus van der Leeuw," *Harvard Divinity School Bulletin* (April 1965), 41.
4. According to Mircea Eliade, "Gerardus van der Leeuw was a versatile genius and a prolific writer . . . Nevertheless, his works do not enjoy the popularity which they deserve. One of the reasons is doubtless his many-sided activities and the *appalling diversity* of his production" (emphasis mine). See "Preface" in Gerardus van der Leeuw, *Sacred and Profane Beauty* (1963), v.
5. See, for example, sociologist Emile Durkheim, *Elementary Forms of Religion* (1995 [1915]) and psychoanalyst Sigmund Freud, *Totem and Taboo* (1950 [1913]), *Future of an Illusion* (1961 [1929]), and *Civilization and Its Discontents* (1961 [1929]).
6. Gerardus van der Leeuw, *Godsvoorstellingen in de oud-Aegyptische pyramideteksten* ("Ideas of God in the Ancient Egyptian Pyramid Texts"), Th.D. dissertation, University of Leiden (1916).
7. "La religion égyptienne a été ainsi mon point de départ que j'ai pris soin de ne jamais perdre de vue." Gerardus van der Leeuw, "Confession Scientifique: Faites à l'Université Masaryk de Bruno, le lundi 18 novembre 1946," *Numen: International Review for the History of Religions* (1954), 9. Hereafter, "CS."
8. CS 10; Waardenburg (1978), 189.
9. Waardenburg (1978), 189-90.
10. Gerardus van der Leeuw, *Inleiding tot de godsdienstgeschiedenis* ("Introduction to the History of Religion") (1924); *Phänomenologie der Religion* (1933); REM xxi. Van der Leeuw made edits to his 1933 text for a French translation made in 1948, *La religion dans son essence et ses manifestations. Phénoménologie de la religion.* This

French text was translated into a second German edition of 1956. Hans Penner relied on this second German edition to translate emendations made to the 1948 text. These emendations are included as appendices in the Princeton translation of the first edition.

11. Jacques Waardenburg, "The Problem of Representing Religions and Religion," in Kippenberg and Luchesi (1991), 42. Waardenburg names other Dutch phenomenologists whose influence permeated this time as: C.P. Tiele (1830-1902), Chantepie de la Saussaye (1848-1920), W.B. Kristensen (1867-1953), C.J. Bleeker (1899-1983), K.A.H. Hidding, Th. P. van Baaren (1912-1989), and F. Sierksma. Saussaye and Kristensen were both teachers of van der Leeuw; Sierksma was his student. See Waardenburg in Kippenberg and Luchesi (1991), 40-1.

12. Waardenburg in Kippenberg and Luchesi (1991), 45.

13. Eric Sharpe, *Comparative Religion* (1986), 229.

14. Von Baaren's essay, published in 1957, was titled, *De ethnologische basis van de Faenomenologie van G. van der Leeuw*. See Lammert Leertouwer, "Gerardus van der Leeuw as a Critic of Culture," Kippenberg and Luchesi (1991), 59.

15. Waardenburg in Kippenberg and Luchesi (1991), 46-7.

16. See J. Waardenburg, "Religion Between Reality and Idea: A Century of Phenomenology of Religion in the Netherlands," *Numen* (1971), 202.

17. Waardenburg in Kippenberg and Luchesi (1991), 54.

18. See Charlotte Allen, "Is Nothing Sacred?" in *Lingua Franca* (1996).

19. Gerardus van der Leeuw, "Some recent achievements of psychological research and their application to history, in particular the history of religions (1926)," in Jacques Waardenburg, *Classical Approaches to the Study of Religion* (1973), 399. Hereafter, "SRA."

20. CS 10. "J'ai toujours plus senti le besoin de trouver un moyen pour embrasser tout ce vaste domaine des religions du monde, sans être restreint aux quelques provinces dont la langue et la civilisation mêétait accessibles et sans pourtant m'égarer dans un dilettantisme mal fondé. Et derrière ce besoin d'orientation et de perspective se faisait sentir de plus en plus fortement le besoin de pénétrer au sein de ce phénomène impressionnant et énigmatique qu'est la religion, de trouver le chemin qui mène des phénomènes épars et quasi détachés des religions historiques à l'essence du phénomene, de procéder des religions à la religion, à son être comme il se montre à nous" (my translation).

21. CS 11-2. Van der Leeuw does propose his own content for the concept of "religion" in the first chapters of his *Religion in Essence and Manifestation*. This definition will be discussed along with that offered in the "Epilogomena" in Chapter 7. Here, I concentrate on how this concept functions in relation to theology and the history of religions.

22. CS 12. "[S]ans la classification, sans le choix, sans la pénétration à l'aide de l'introspection qui font dans leur ensemble la méthode phénoménologique" (my translation).

23. Hubbeling describes how van der Leeuw tempered the young Hubbeling's empirical proclivities by teaching him that he has to identify something as religious before he can begin to describe it. See Hubbeling, H.G. *Divine Presence in Ordinary Life: Gerardus van der Leeuw's twofold method in his thinking on art and religion* (1986), 4.
24. While van der Leeuw uses "theology" as a generic term, capable of referring to traditions other than his own, when speaking as a theologian, it is always as a Christian theologian.
25. Quoted from van der Leeuw, *Inleiding tot de theologie* ("Introduction to Theology") (1948), 106-8, in Carman (1965), 21.
26. *Inleiding*, 234-6; Carman (1965), 23-4.
27. Ibid.
28. *Inleiding*, 233; Carman (1965), 23.
29. CS 13. "Je n'ai jamais éprouvé le besoin d'oublier que je suis théologien, et naturellement j'ai cherché à faire profiter la théologie de la methode phenomenologique. Non pas, assurement, pour faire de la théologie une science de la religion, mais au contraire pour faire mieux ressortir la méthode théologique qui, de mon avis, est absolument autonome . . . Or, la phénoménologie doit aider la théologie à grouper les fait, à en pénétrer le sens, à en trouver l'essence, avant qu'elle puisse les évaluer et les employer pour ses fins dogmatiques" (my translation).
30. Carman (1965), 27.
31. The distinction among these three disciplines is slippery, as historians may study theological proclamations as case material, and theologians may assert the "truth" of "historical" facts. This is van der Leeuw's point. No member of this braid is ever absent in any moment in which a person attends to religion: historical facts, phenomenological understanding, and theological assumptions are always all at play in the relationship between the religionist and religion.
32. Carman (1965), 41.

6: A Practice of Understanding

1. Gerardus van der Leeuw, "On Phenomenology and Its Relation to Theology (1928)," in Waardenburg (1973), 407. Hereafter, "OPR."
2. REM 671-95; in particular, Chapter 107, "Phenomenon and Phenomenology," 671-8. For my analyses of the Epilogomena, I rely on the English translation of the 1932 edition approved by van der Leeuw. In the Epilogomena, chapters on "religion" and "the phenomenology of religion" succeed a chapter on "the phenomenon and phenomenology." Although this organization of chapters might seem to suggest an interpretation of van der Leeuw's work that I have rejected—namely, that method precedes the object to which it is applied—the Epilogomena as a whole appears as a footnote to a long

treatise on religion. Thus, its placement in the text qualifies its internal arrangement: phenomenology is always already steeped in the forms of religions.

3. In the choice of the term "practice," I indirectly engage recent work among anthropologists and sociologists [e.g., Bourdieu (1977); de Certeau (1984); Bell (1992, 1997)], and suggest parallels that warrant exploration beyond the pages of this book.

4. Wim Hofstee points out in "The French Connection: Gerardus van der Leeuw and the Concept of Primitive Mentality" [in Kippenberg and Luchesi (1991), 127-137], that discussions concerning "influence" on van der Leeuw are "fruitless" given his vast correspondence and extensive reading. Even terms he lifts from other disciplines are mediated and elaborated by his reading in other fields. Such is the case for his definition of "understanding," or *Verstehen*, as imaginative empathy, which he gleans from his reading in structural psychology— in particular, Jaspers, Spranger, and Dilthey. See REM 678, for bibliographic references.

5. Here van der Leeuw's approach to theory and method finds a contemporary echo in Geertz's call for a theory that is close to the ground in his *The Interpretation of Cultures* (1973), Chapter 1.

6. Van der Leeuw mentions Husserl once in the Epilegomena to mention that he also used the word "*epoche*." Yet van der Leeuw proceeds to define the word with reference to structural psychologists and the conditions necessary for imaginative empathy; he also references Schleiermacher, Hegel, and Kierkegaard. Waardenburg criticizes Ninian Smart for claiming in his "Introduction" to *Religion in Essence and Manifestation* (van der Leeuw, 1996) that Husserl was a formative influence on van der Leeuw. Others agree with Waardenburg. See Waardenburg (1971), 171, 201; Kippenberg and Luchesi (1991), 44, 129, 131; Sharpe (1986), 223; Hubbeling (1986), 7.

7. This argument is repeated among contemporary theorists as well. Victor Turner will critique Sigmund Freud as too "theological" for making a determination that "gods . . . are creations of the human mind" [*Totem and Taboo* (1950 [1913]), 24]. In Turner's words, Freud takes up the "implicitly theological position of trying to explain, or explain away, religious phenomena as the product of psychological or sociological causes" [*The Ritual Process* (1995 [1966]), 4].

8. Van der Leeuw, "On Understanding (1935)," in Waardenburg (1973), 410. Hereafter, "OU."

9. REM 688-9. Quoted from *Begrebet Angest*, "The Concept of Dread."

10. The use of play as a concept in the study of culture is generally attributed to Johan Huizinga, van der Leeuw's fellow countryman and frequent correspondent. See Huizinga (1938); and Y.B. Kuiper, "The

Primitive and the Past: van der Leeuw and Huizinga as Critics of
Culture," in Kippenberg and Luchesi (1991), 113-125.

11. REM 675. It is interesting to read van der Leeuw alongside the
participant-observer model of ethnology being developed by his
contemporary, Bronislav Malinowski. Van der Leeuw urges the
utmost degree of empathy, practiced at a distance, while participant-
observation involves objective reporting at close range. See Sharpe
(1986), 176, 235. For a contemporary discussion, see Clifford Geertz,
Works and Lives (1988), 83ff.

7: Understanding Religion and Dance

1. Isadora Duncan (1879-1927) was one of the first Americans to earn
international acclaim for her "interpretive" dances. She toured and
lived in Europe from 1900 until her death, taking brief excursions to
the United States and South America. She considered the Netherlands
her "fine little Holland country," toured there often, and went there to
birth her first child. Van der Leeuw would have had the opportunity to
see her as a teenager, while studying in Germany (1915-16), or again
in Holland in 1921. See Lillian Loewenthal, "Isadora Duncan in the
Netherlands," 1979-1980, 227-253. One of van der Leeuw's plates
(#45) in *Paths and Boundaries* is a drawing of Duncan. For a discussion
of Duncan's influence on van der Leeuw, see LaMothe, "Why Dance?

2. In *Sacred and Profane Beauty: The Holy in Art* (1963), van der Leeuw
admits that his own denomination, the Geregromeerde, was even
more resistant to dance than other Protestant and Catholic
Christianities (S 1-2; W 65). *Sacred and Profane Beauty* will hereafter
be refered to as "S" and *Wegen en Grenzen* (1948) will hereafter will
be refered to as "W."

3. Gerardus van der Leeuw, *In den hemel is enen dance.* (1930); "*In dem
Himmel ist ein Tanz . . . Uber dies religiose Bedeutung des Tanzes*"
und des Festzuges (1931) ("'In heaven there is a Dance . . .' On the
religious meaning of dance and festival.").

4. Between 1932 and 1948, van der Leeuw "fundamentally changed" the
framework of the original and doubled its size (Hubbeling 1986, 24-5).
Where the first edition was organized according to phenomenological
structures organizing historical relationships between art and religion,
the second edition was organized by the arts themselves, with
phenomenological structures appearing as subheadings beneath each
art. Although Hubbeling laments the subordination of the structures
to the arts, I suggest that this change accommodates van der Leeuw's
increasing conviction that theological proclamation is both enabled and
deflected by phenomenological understanding. Hubbeling admits that
van der Leeuw was increasingly convinced that human knowledge of

God is inevitably and necessarily mediated by symbols and sacraments (Hubbeling 1986, 22). By arranging his historical materials by art rather than phenomenological structure, then, van der Leeuw allows himself a greater degree of flexibility in discussing the manner in which each type of art mediates religious experience—even as he admits that the divisions among the arts themselves are fluid and culturally specific.

5. It is impossible to invoke the concept of power without alluding to the work of Michel Foucault. Foucault and van der Leeuw share a view of power as productive, active over a network of particular points, carried out through the movement of human bodies; they both see individuals as effects of power. Van der Leeuw places a greater emphasis on human agency. A detailed comparison would be worthwhile. See Foucault, *Power/Knowledge* (1980). Van der Leeuw's use of the term was influenced by concepts like *mana, orenda,* and *wakanda* current among the theories of dynamism and animism he otherwise rejected (Waardenberg [1971], 162).

6. Note that what appears to a scholar as religious may or may not be perceived by involved individuals as religious, or as pertaining to a given religion. Van der Leeuw's task is to determine what characterizes those moments when a scholar experiences and names another's experience of something as religion. This process may or may not correspond with the terms another person uses to describe what he is doing. Then again, if a person did describe his action as "religion," his description would be a "sign" warranting interpretation.

7. Foucault 1980.

8. For a discussion of these dynamics, see Judith Butler, *The Psychic Life of Power* (1997).

9. Such a critique of ritual theory and theorists has been eloquently made by Catherine Bell in *Ritual Theory, Ritual Practice* (1992).

10. S 6; W 5. Van der Leeuw stresses this point with a selective use of capital letters for Beauty and Holiness as entities versus beauty and holiness as human experiences. This point is lost across the translations into German (where all nouns are capitalized) and then English (where nouns are selectively capitalized).

11. These sentences allude to the history of aesthetics in the modern West whose formative moment is often traced to the third critique of Immanuel Kant, *Critique of Judgment* (1987). In this critique, Kant argues that aesthetic judgment is a faculty of human cognition. He identifies aesthetic judgment with a feeling of beauty which arises when the sensuous form of an object corresponds with the concepts and structures of human reason. Kant's analysis defines the terms within which the history of modern aesthetics has unfolded.

12. For how far away such recognition fell in the American Christian context, see Ann Wagner's *Adversaries of Dance: From the Puritans to the Present* (1997).

13. This reading does not fully immure van der Leeuw from critiques of essentialism. It still may be argued that the concepts of art and religion are hopelessly informed by western understandings of these terms. Van der Leeuw would probably agree, and then acknowledge that one must begin somewhere. R. J. Zwi Werblowsky remembers how van der Leeuw would say, "if you want to collect facts, you better collect stamps"(Werblowsky, 147 in Kippenberg and Luchesi [1991]).

14. Gerardus van der Leeuw, *Wegen en Grenzen. Studie over de verhouding van religie en kunst,* 1955 ("Paths and Boundaries: Reflections on the Relationship between Religion and Art"). Hereafter, "W 55." For this edition, Smelik rearranged paragraphs (and sometimes pages) of the text, changed some section titles and added others, omitted van der Leeuw's 1948 *"Voorrede voor den Tweeden Druk"* ("Foreword for the Second Edition"), and contributed one of his own. Nevertheless, for the most part, the structure of the book follows van der Leeuw's 1948 rendition.

15. Gerardus van der Leeuw, *Vom Heiligen und der Kunst* (1957) ("The Holy and Art"), translated by Frau Dr. Annelotte Piper. Hereafter, "VHK."

16. While the German and English translations hew closely to the text of Smelik's edition, they also depart from it at significant moments. Moreover, both of these translations delete all page references from van der Leeuw's footnotes and fail to reproduce the 85 plates and ten fragments of musical compositions that van der Leeuw included as illustrations at the end of his text.

17. In my study of the text(s), I rely on Green's English translation of Smelik's third edition, which I check against the organization and original Dutch of van der Leeuw's 1948 version. Where significant differences appear between the 1948 Dutch edition and the English translation, I examine Smelik's 1955 edition and its German translation in order to discern in whose hands the changes occurred.

18. See Leertouwer in Kippenberg and Luchesi (1991), 62.

19. See R.J. Zwi Werblowsky, "Between 'Primitive' and 'Modern'," in Kippenberg and Luchesi (1991), 141-8.

20. Here again, reading van der Leeuw through the work of his editors is challenging. Smelik, in the edition he published after van der Leeuw's death, created the category of "The Dance and Contemporary Culture," placed the category at the end of van der Leeuw's chapter on "Beautiful Movement," and gathered van der Leeuw's discussions regarding dance and the "modern" under it. In so doing, Smelik's edition gives the

impression that van der Leeuw is espousing an evolutionary progress from primitive to modern—a progression that van der Leeuw's earlier organization explicitly rejected.

21. In so doing, he also anticipates contemporary critiques of intellectual colonialism. See David Chidester (1996); Asad (1993); Marianna Torgovnick (1990), and the classic, Edward Said's *Orientalism* (1978) for examples and critiques of intellectual colonialism.

22. S 7; W 6. From this point forward, I use the word primitive without quotation marks to refer to van der Leeuw's phenomenological structure—that is, to the kinds of social and psychological organization which appear to him as "primitive."

23. On the relation of van der Leeuw to Levy-Bruhl and his notion of the primitive, see Wim Hofstee, "The French Connection: Gerardus van der Leeuw and the Concept of Primitive Mentality," in Kippenberg and Luchesi (1991), 127-37. In his anti-evolutionist stance, van der Leeuw followed in the footsteps of Franz Boas, whose 1911 *The Mind of Primitive Man* sounded an early note of cultural relativism. On Western views of the primitive, see Torgovnick (1990).

24. S 7; W 6. As with the German *Geist*, the Dutch *geeste* means both "mind" and "spirit," thereby defying translation into English. When combined with *structur*, the resulting word references the intellectual, religious, psychological, and social forms that define and represent a given human culture.

25. S 9; W 7. Van der Leeuw uses two words which are translated as "movement" or "motion": *"beweging"* which, as a verbal noun, is closer to "movement"; and *"gang"* which is closer to "motion," in the sense of a general flurry of activity. The English translation is not consistent in its translation of these terms. In the majority of cases, van der Leeuw uses *"beweging"* to refer to the movement of something, a stylized or ordered motion, while *"gang"* suggests motion in general. Thus, dance, as *schoone beweging* ("beautiful movement") is also *geordende gang* ("ordered motion"). I follow this usage.

26. Of the other arts, music ranks a close second. Van der Leeuw introduces the five structures plus theological aesthetics, yet must qualify the antithetical structure to accommodate music because Christianity has not manifested a full-blown conflict with music in general—only with particular forms of it.

8: Spinning the Unity of Life: Dance as Religion

1. Van der Leeuw was not a feminist. He does not address the question of whose body he is describing. Yet all the examples he gives for the dances described indiscriminately include dances performed by men, by women, and by both together.

2. For a contemporary exploration of dance as mobilizing the "lived body" of human experience, see Sondra Horton Fraleigh, *Dance and the Lived Body: A Descriptive Aesthetics* (1987).
3. Victor Turner, Richard Schechner, and others develop the notion of "reflexivity" in order to talk about "performance" as a category for social analysis. I use the term with reference to bodily movement specifically. I aim to find a way to articulate the agency of bodily being in religious life against those who would emphasize its passivity. Too often a ritual dance is described as inscribing "the body" or embedding social codes. See essays in *By Means of Performance* (1990), edited by Richard Schechner and Willa Appel. For critique, see LaMothe, "Why Dance?"
4. For an alternative discussion of this logic, see Kimerer L. LaMothe, "Giving Birth to a Dancing Star," *Soundings* (2003).
5. The term "culture" emerged in scholarly discourse at the turn of the century as a vehicle for critiquing perceived changes in western civilization and for participating consciously in its future development. Van der Leeuw held that religion served as the basis for all cult or culture; in theological terms, culture is the name for the human activity that occurs between Creation and Recreation. Leertouwer, for one, identifies van der Leeuw's phenomenology of religion as an attempt to engage creatively and critically in the activity of culture of which it is a part. See Leertouwer in Kippenberg and Luchesi (1991), 57-63. See Raymond Williams, *Culture and Society* (1958); Geertz (1973); and for a contemporary critiques, Adam Kuper, *Culture* (1999).
6. In choosing the Dutch *beschaving* van der Leeuw rejects the the germanic *cultuur*, emphasizing culture as a process of creation and movement.
7. Here van der Leeuw approaches Durkheim's conception of society: culture is the process in which human beings symbolize the community of which they are members. See Durkheim, *The Elementary Forms of Religious Life* (1995).
8. With this association of culture with embodied movement, van der Leeuw sidesteps the current controversy over the relation of conflicting and overlapping symbolic universes. In the process of meaning-making that culture is, the universes are the material on which a person draws in order to respond to her experiences. For an account of these controversies, see Kuper (1999).
9. See Maxine Sheets-Johnstone, *The Roots of Thinking* (1990), for a contemporary account of how bodily movement serves as the medium in and through which humans learn language and become participants in culture.

10. Debate continues to rage whether or not it is possible to define a kind of movement that is "natural" to humans, or whether every basic human movement is always already informed by the cultural and experiential contexts in which an individual grows. See Judith Lynne Hanna, *To Dance Is Human* (1987), Chapter 2, for a summary of this debate. The phrase van der Leeuw uses to describe movement other than dance is not "natural" (as translated), but *reilt en zeilt,* a Dutch idiom meaning the usual or ordinary. Van der Leeuw explains that dance is not learned movement per se, but movement which represents a particular consciousness or intentionality of a human in relation to himself and the world.

11. S 289; W 278. Though translated as "act of aggression," van der Leeuw's *verovering* carries less of a negative emotional content and assures a victory or mastery which "act of aggression" does not.

12. This analysis does not preclude the fact that success is not always guaranteed, that a ritual can fail and people lose faith. It does provide an explanation of why rituals can endure many "failures" before such a crisis occurs. For a classic case of a failed ritual, see Geertz (1973), Chapter 6.

13. S 16; W 15. Here *schakelt* conveys a sense of "gearing" or "engagement" as gears come together to enable a transfer of power.

14. See Susan Foster, *Reading Dancing* (1986), for an excellent account of how different forms of movement make different kinds of bodies.

15. S 29; W 27. In the 1948 and 1955 Dutch editions, this quotation appears in a footnote.

16. For the positions pro and con, see Backman (1952) and Davies (1984) respectively.

17. S 253; W 419-20. "Beweging—en die is in alle kunst essentieel," my translation.

18. Van der Leeuw was not the first nor the last to make use of this idea. It is most frequently associated with evolutionary theories of language, religion, and culture. See R.G. Collingwood, *The Principles of Art* (1938), for an example of an evolutionary perspective; see Suzanne Langer (1953) for a critique that is friendly to dance, though less so to religion.

19. S 79, my italics; W 106-7.

20. S 226; W 384. "De muziek is een groote worsteling om het 'gansch Andere' te bereiken, dat zij toch nimmer kan uitdrukken." "Music is a great struggle to reach the 'wholly Other' which it can never express."

21. S 329; W 466. Here *gestremde* conveys a sense of "dammed," "congealed," or "coagulated." Note that Green translates *gestremde* using the same word that he uses elsewhere to translate *verstarde* in relation to dance, namely, "petrified."

9: Marking Boundaries: Dance against Religion

1. Van der Leeuw's use of the term "fossil" or "survival" recalls James Frazer in *The Golden Bough* (1890) when he uses the term to describe traces of the "savage" left in modern ideas and images. However, while Frazer identified the primitive as a historical category and sought to find in it the "universal truth about human nature," van der Leeuw appeals to the primitive as a phenomenological category, not bound by chronology. See discussion in Torgovick (1990), 7.
2. See discussion above, chapter 7, pp. 201-202.
3. For a description of hostility towards dance in the context of American Christianity, see Wagner (1997).
4. How this fall correlates with the development of asceticism, monasticism, and church authority/unity as expressions of Christian faith demands further research and attention. See Davies (1984); M.F. Taylor (1967).
5. S 55; W 69. Whether or not this description accurately describes early Christianity continues to occupy scholars of religion. See Margaret Miles, *Fullness of Life: Historical Foundations for a New Asceticism* (1981); Peter Brown, *Body and Society* (1988); and Carolyn Walker Bynum, *The Resurrection of the Body in Western Christianity, 200-1336* (1995).
6. S 66; W 88. From Emil Utitz, *Der Kunstler*, Stuttgart (1925).

Conclusion to Part 2: Can Dance Be Religion?

1. Foucault (1980), 128-9.
2. Foucault (1980), 81-2.

10: Dancing Religion

1. Does this claim hold true even in the case of a purely rational religion? I believe so. A purely rational religion is a philosophy. Why call it religion at all? If the intent is to imply that one's philosophy performs the same function as claims to supernatural beings, for example, then the very use of the term in this way proves the statement true. To name some nexus of culture as religion is to notice some effect of power or transformation that makes a difference for someone. The nature of that power and the difference it makes is what the field exists to debate.
2. This literature is extensive. See works in the bibliography by: Linda Nicholson, Grace Jantzen, Luce Irigaray, Julia Kristeva, Judith Butler, Seyla Benhabib, G. Lloyd. See also work by Friedrich Nietzsche, Michel Foucault, Jacques Derrida, Mark C. Taylor, and John Caputo.
3. The preoccupation with "the body" is evident in work which builds on the theories of bodily practice leveled by Pierre Bourdieu, Michel

de Certeau, Michel Foucault, and Catherine Bell; on theories of gender, performance and performativity as developed most notably by Judith Butler; on historical explorations into lived religion and material culture; and on volumes such as Sarah Coakley's *Religion and the Body* (1997).

4. Currents of thought represented by Michel Foucault, Jacques Lacan, respectively, and their followers and critics. See Judith Butler, *The Psychic Life of Power* (1997) for discussion.

5. See Adams and Apostolos-Cappadona (1990) for a representative sampling of the field. See also Judith Rock (1978); Rock and Mealy (1988); J. G. Davies (1984); Taylor (1967); Gagne et al, (1999).

Bibliography

Philosophy and Theology

Bacon, Francis. *Works 1622–3*, vol II. Collected and edited by James Spedding, Robert L. Ellis, and Douglas D. Heath. New York: Garrett Press, 1968.

Beiser, Frederick, ed. *Cambridge Companion to Hegel*. Cambridge, UK: Cambridge University Press, 1993.

Benhabib, Seyla. *Situating the Self: Gender, Community and Postmodernism in Contemporary Ethics*. New York: Routledge, 1992.

Buber, Martin. *I and Thou*. Tr. Walter Kaufmann. New York: Simon & Schuster, 1996.

Butler, Judith. *The Psychic Life of Power*. Stanford: Stanford University Press, 1997.

———. *Bodies That Matter: On the Discursive Limits of Sex*. New York: Routledge, 1993.

———. *Gender Trouble*. New York: Routledge, 1990.

Caputo, John. *More Radical Hermeneutics: On Not Knowing Who We Are*. Bloomington, IN: Indiana University Press, 2000.

Cavell, Stanley. *Philosophical Passages*. Cambridge, UK: Blackwell Publishers, 1995.

———. *The Claim of Reason: Wittgenstein, Skepticism, Morality and Tragedy*. New York: Oxford University Press, 1979.

Certeau, Michel de. *The Practice of Everyday Life*. Tr. Steven Rendall. Berkeley, CA: University of California Press, 1984.

Cixous, Hélène. "The Laugh of the Medusa." 245-264 in *New French Feminisms*. Eds. Elaine Marks and Isabelle de Courtivron. New York: Schocken Books, 1981.

Clarke, Eric O. "Fetal Attraction: Hegel's An-aesthetics of Gender." 149-175 in *Feminist Interpretations of G.W.F. Hegel.*, Ed. Patricia J. Mills. University Park, PA: Pennsylvania State University Press, 1996.

Coakley, Sarah, ed. *Religion and the Body*. Cambridge, UK: Cambridge University Press, 1997.

Collingwood, R.G. *The Principles of Art*. London: Oxford University Press, 1938.

Daly, Mary. *Gyn/Ecology: The Metaethics of Radical Feminism*. Boston: Beacon Press, 1978.

Descartes, René. *Discourse on Method and Meditations on First Philosophy*. Ed. David Weissman. New Haven: Yale University Press, 1996.

———. *Discourse on Method*. Tr. Laurence J. Lafleur. New York: Macmillan, 1956 [1637].

Derrida, Jacques. *Of Grammatology*. Tr. Gayatri Spivak. Baltimore, MD: Johns Hopkins University Press, 1976.

Derrida, Jacques, and Christie V. McDonald. "Choreographies." *Diacritics* 12, no. 2: 66-76.

Eagleton, Terry. *The Ideology of the Aesthetic*. Oxford: Blackwell Publishers, 1990.

Feuerbach, Ludwig. *The Essence of Christianity*. Tr. George Eliot. New York: Harper Torchbooks, 1957 [1841].

Forster, Michael N. *Hegel's Idea of a Phenomenology of Spirit*. Chicago: University of Chicago Press, 1998.

Foucault, Michel. "What Is Enlightenment?" 32-50 in *Foucault Reader*, ed. P. Rabinow. New York: Pantheon Books, 1984.

———. *Power/Knowledge: Selected Interviews and Other Writings 1972-1977*. Ed./Tr. Colin Gordon. New York: Random House, Pantheon Books, 1980.

———. *Discipline and Punish: The Birth of the Prison*. Tr. Alan Sheridan. New York: Vintage Books, 1977.

———. *The Order of Things: An Archeology of the Human Sciences*. New York: Vintage Books, 1973.

Freud, Sigmund. *Civilization and Its Discontents*. Tr. James Strachey. New York: W.W. Norton, 1961 [1929].

Gay, Peter. *The Enlightenment: An Interpretation, Volume II: The Science of Freedom*. New York: Norton, 1969.

Gerrish, Brian. *A Prince of the Church: Schleiermacher and the Beginnings of Modern Theology*. Philadelphia: Fortress Press, 1984.

Jantzen, Grace. *Becoming Divine: Toward a Feminist Philosophy of Religion*. Bloomington, IN: Indiana University Press, 1999.

———. *Power, Gender and Mysticism*. Cambridge, UK: Cambridge University Press, 1995.

Habermas, Jurgen. *The Structural Transformation of the Public Sphere*. Cambridge, MA: MIT Press, 1989.

Hardy, Edward, ed. *Christology of the Later Fathers*. Philadelphia: Westminster Press, 1954.

Hegel, G.W.F. *Lectures on the Philosophy of Religion, 1827.* Ed. Peter Hodgson. Berkeley, CA: University of California Press, 1988.

———. *Phänomenologie des Geistes.* Hamburg: Felix Meiner, 1988.

———. *Phenomenology of Spirit.* Tr. A.V. Miller. New York: Oxford University Press, 1977 [1806].

Heyward, Carter. *Touching Our Strength: The Erotic as Power and the Love of God.* New York: Harper Collins, 1989.

Hollywood, Amy. *Sensible Ecstasy: Mysticism, Sexual Difference, and the Demands of History.* Chicago: University of Chicago Press, 2002.

Huizinga, Johan. *Homo Ludens: A Study of the Play Element in Culture.* Boston: Beacon Press, 1950 [1938].

Hutchings, Kimberly. *Hegel and Feminist Philosophy.* Oxford: Blackwell Publishers, 2003.

Irigaray, Luce. *Sexes and Genealogies.* Tr. Gillian Gill. New York: Columbia University Press, 1993 [1987].

———. *Speculum of the Other Woman.* Tr. Gillian Gill. Ithaca, NY: Cornell University Press, 1985.

Kant, Immanuel. *Kant's Political Writings.* Tr. H.B. Nisbet. Cambridge, UK: Cambridge University Press, 1991.

———. *Critique of Judgement.* Tr. W.S. Pluhar. Indianapolis: Hackett Publishing Co., 1987 [1793].

———. *Critique of Practical Reason.* Tr. Lewis White Beck. New York: Macmillan, 1985 [1788].

———. *Critique of Pure Reason.* Tr. Norman Kemp Smith. New York: St. Martin's Press, 1965 [1787].

———. *Religion within the Limits of Reason Alone.* Tr. Theodore Greene & Hoyt Hudson. New York: Harper Torchbooks, 1960 [1793].

Kaufman, Gordon. *In Face of Mystery.* Cambridge, MA: Harvard University Press, 1993.

Kierkegaard, Søren. *Concluding Unscientific Postscript to "Philosophical Fragments."* Volumes I and II. Eds./Trs. Howard Hong and Edna Hong. Princeton: Princeton University Press, 1992 [1846].

———. *Fear and Trembling and Repetition.* Trs. Howard Hong and Edna Hong. Princeton: Princeton University Press, 1983 [1843].

Kristeva, Julia. *Powers of Horror: An Essay on Abjection.* Tr. Leon S. Roudriez. New York: Columbia University Press, 1982.

———. *Desire in Language: A Semiotic Approach to Literature and Art.* Trs. T. Gora, A. Jardine, L.S. Roudiez. New York: Columbia University Press, 1980.

Lacoue-Labarthe, Philippe, and Jean-Luc Nancy. *The Literary Absolute: The Theory of Literature in German Romanticism.* Albany, NY: SUNY Press, 1988.

LaMothe, Kimerer L. "Reason, Religion, and Sexual Difference: Resources for a Feminist Philosophy of Religion in Hegel's *Phenomenology of Spirit*." *Hypatia* 2, no. 2 (Summer 2005).

——. "Giving Birth to a Dancing Star: Reading Friedrich Nietzsche's Maternal Rhetoric via Isadora Duncan's Dance." *Soundings*. Vol. LXXXVI, No. 3–4. Fall/Winter 2003.

Langer, Susanne K. *Feeling and Form*. New York: Charles Scribner's Sons, 1953.

Leder, Drew. *The Absent Body*. Chicago: University of Chicago Press, 1990.

Léon, Céline, and Sylvia Walsh, eds. *Feminist Interpretations of Søren Kierkegaard*. University Park, PA: Pennsylvania State University Press, 1997.

Lloyd, Genevieve. *The Man of Reason*. Minneapolis: University of Minnesota Press, 1984.

Lowrie, Walter. *A Short Life of Kierkegaard*. Princeton: Princeton University Press, 1970 [1942].

Marion, Jean Luc. *On Descartes' Metaphysical Prism: The Constitution and the Limits of Onto-theo-logy in Cartesian Thought*. Tr. Jeffrey L. Kosky. Chicago: University of Chicago Press, 1999.

Marks, Elaine, and Isabelle de Courtivron, eds. *New French Feminisms*. New York: Schocken Books, 1981.

Matustik, Martin, and Merold Westphal, eds. *Kierkegaard in Post/Modernity*. Bloomington, IN: Indiana University Press, 1995.

McCloskey, Mary A. *Kant's Aesthetics*. New York: SUNY Press, 1997.

Merleau-Ponty, Maurice. *The Merleau-Ponty Aesthetics Reader: Philosophy and Painting*. Ed./Tr. Galen A. Johnson. Evanston, IL: Northwestern University Press, 1993.

——. *Signs*. Tr. Richard C. McCleary. Evanston, IL: Northwestern University Press, 1964.

——. *Phenomenology of Perception*. Tr. Colin Smith. London: Routledge & Kegan Paul, 1962.

Mills, Patricia Jagentowicz, ed. *Feminist Interpretations of G.W.F. Hegel*. University Park, PA: Pennsylvania State University Press, 1996.

Nancy, Jean-Luc. *Hegel: The Restlessness of the Negative*. Trs. Jason Smith and Steven Miller. Minneapolis: University of Minnesota Press, 2002.

Nelson, James B. *Embodiment: An Approach to Sexuality and Christian Theology*. Minneapolis: Augsburg Press, 1978.

Neuhouser, Frederick. *Foundations of Hegel's Social Theory: Actualizing Freedom*. Cambridge, MA: Harvard University Press, 2000.

Nicholson, Linda. *The Play of Reason*. Ithaca, NY: Cornell University Press, 1999.

Nietzsche, Friedrich. *The Birth of Tragedy and the Case of Wagner*. Tr. Walter Kaufmann. New York: Vintage Books, 1967.

———. *The Genealogy of Morals and Ecce Homo.* Trs. Walter Kaufmann and R.J. Hollingdale. New York: Vintage Books, 1967.

———. *The Portable Nietzsche.* Tr./Ed. Walter Kaufmann. New York: Viking Press, 1954.

Oliver, Kelly. *Witnessing: Beyond Recognition.* Minneapolis: University of Minnesota Press, 2001.

Pinkard, Terry. *Hegel's Phenomenology: The Sociality of Reason.* Cambridge, UK: Cambridge University Press, 1994.

Pippin, Robert. *Hegel's Idealism: The Satisfactions of Self-Consciousness.* Cambridge, UK: Cambridge University Press, 1995.

Proudfoot, Wayne. *Religious Experience.* Berkeley, CA: University of California, 1985.

Richardson, Ruth D. *The Role of Women in the Life and Thoughts of Early Schleiermacher (1768-1806).* Lewiston, NY: Edwin Mellen Press, 1991.

Ruether, Rosemary Radford. *Sexism and God-Talk: Toward a Feminist Theology.* Boston: Beacon Press, 1983.

Schleiermacher, Friedrich. *The Christian Faith.* Ed. H. R. Mackintosh and J. S. Stewart. Edinburgh: T&T Clark, 1989 [1821].

———. *On Religion: Speeches to Its Cultured Despisers.* Ed. Richard Crouter. Cambridge, UK: Cambridge University Press. 1988.

Sheets-Johnstone, Maxine. *The Primacy of Movement.* Amsterdam, Philadelphia: John Benjamins Publishing, 1999.

———. *The Roots of Thinking.* Philadelphia: Temple University Press, 1990.

Stewart, Jon, ed. *The Hegel Myths and Legends.* Evanston, IL: Northwestern University, 1996.

Taylor, Charles. *Sources of the Self: The Making of the Modern Identity.* Cambridge, MA: Harvard University Press, 1989.

———. *Hegel.* Cambridge, UK: Cambridge University Press, 1975.

Taylor, Mark C. *Disfiguring: Art, Architecture, Religion.* Chicago: University of Chicago Press, 1992.

———. *Altarity.* Chicago: University of Chicago Press, 1987.

———. *Erring: A Postmodern A/theology.* Chicago: University of Chicago Press, 1984.

———. *Journeys to Selfhood: Hegel and Kierkegaard.* Berkeley, CA: University of California Press, 1980.

Tillich, Paul. *Systematic Theology: Volume Three.* Chicago: University of Chicago Press, 1959.

Twiss, Sumner, and Walter Conser, Jr., eds. *Experience of the Sacred: Readings in the Phenomenology of Religion.* Hanover, NH: Brown University Press, 1992.

Utitz, Emil. *Der Kunstler.* Stuttgart, 1925.

Westphal, Merold. *History and Truth in Hegel's Phenomenology.* Bloomington, IN: Indiana University Press, 1998.

Williams, Raymond. *Culture and Society 1880-1950*. London: Chatto & Windus, Ltd., 1958.

Wittgenstein, Ludwig. *Philosophical Investigations*. Tr. G.E.M. Anscombe. New York: MacMillan, 1958.

Wollstonecraft, Mary. A Vindication of the Rights of Woman. New York: Everyman's Library, 1992 [1792].

Religious Studies, Anthropology, and Critical Theory

Allen, Charlotte. "Is Nothing Sacred?" *Lingua Franca* (November 1996): 30-40.

Almond, Philip C. *The British Discovery of Buddhism*. Cambridge, UK: Cambridge University Press, 1988.

Asad, Talal. *Genealogies of Religion: Discipline and Reasons of Power in Christianity and Islam*. Baltimore, MD: Johns Hopkins Press, 1993.

Bell, Catherine. *Ritual: Perspectives and Dimensions*. New York: Oxford University Press, 1997.

———. "Modernism and Postmodernism in the Study of Religion." *Religious Studies Review* 22, no. 3 (July 1996): 179-190.

———. *Ritual Theory, Ritual Practice*. New York: Oxford University Press, 1992.

Blacking, John. *How Musical is Man?* Seattle: University of Washington Press, 1973.

Boas, Franz. *The Mind of Primitive Man*. New York: Free Press, 1965 [1911].

Bourdieu, Pierre. *Outline of a Theory of Practice*. Tr. Richard Nice. Cambridge, UK: Cambridge University Press, 1977.

Bourguinon, Erica. *Possession*. San Francisco: Chandler & Sharp, 1976.

———. *Trance Dance*. New York: Dance Perspectives Foundation, 1968.

Buckley, Jorunn Jacobsen and Thomas Buckley. "Response: Anthropology, History of Religions, and a Cognitive Approach to Religious Phenomena ." *Journal of the American Academy of Religion* 63, no. 2: 343-352.

Capps, Walter H. *The Making of a Discipline*. Minneapolis: Fortress Press, 1995.

Chidester, David. *Savage Systems: Colonialism and Comparative Religion in Southern Africa*. Charlottesville, VA: University of Virginia Press, 1996.

Durkheim, Emile. *The Elementary Forms of Religious Life*. Tr. Karen E. Fields. New York: The Free Press. 1995.

Frazer, James. *The Golden Bough*. Third edition. London: Macmillan, 1935 [1890].

Freud, Sigmund. *The Future of an Illusion*. Tr. James Strachey. New York: W.W. Norton, 1961.

———. *Totem and Taboo*. Tr. James Strachey. New York: W.W. Norton, 1950.

Geertz, Clifford. *The Interpretation of Cultures.* New York: Basic Books, 1973.
———. *Works and Lives: The Anthropologist as Author.* Stanford, CA: Stanford University Press, 1988.
Gill, Sam. "No Place to Stand: Jonathan Z. Smith as *Homo Ludens,* The Academic Study of Religion *Sub Specie Ludi.*" *Journal of the American Academy of Religion* 66, no. 2: 283-312.
Grimes, Ronald, ed. *Readings in Ritual Studies.* Upper Saddle River, NJ: Prentice Hall, 1996.
Hart, Ray L. "Religious and Theological Studies in American Higher Education: A Pilot Study." *Journal of the American Academy of Religion* 59, no. 4: 715-827.
King, Ursala. "Review Essay: Impasse and Resolution." *Journal of the American Academy of Religion* 61, no. 4: 785-92.
Kuper, Adam. Culture: *The Anthropologists' Account.* Cambridge: Harvard University Press, 1999.
LaMothe, Kimerer L. "Why Dance? Towards a Theory of Religion as Practice and Performance." Unpublished manuscript based on a presentation given at the Center for the Study of World Religions, Harvard University, October 30, 2003.
Lawson, E. Thomas, and Robert N. McCauley. *Rethinking Religion: Connecting Cognition and Culture.* Cambridge, UK: Cambridge University Press, 1990.
———. "Rejoinder: Caring for the Details: A Humane Reply to Buckley and Buckley." *Journal of the American Academy of Religion* 63, no. 2: 353-357.
———. "Crisis of Conscience, Riddle of Identity: Making a Space for a Cognitive Approach to Religious Phenomena." *Journal of the American Academy of Religion* 61, no. 2: 201-223.
MacAloon, John, ed. *Rite, Drama, Festival, Spectacle: Rehearsals Toward a Theory of Cultural Performance.* Philadelphia: Institute for the Study of Human Issues, 1984.
Marret, R. R. *Faith, Hope, and Charity in Primitive Religion.* 1932.
Masuzawa, Tomoko. *In Search of Dreamtime: The Quest for the Origin of Religion.* Chicago: University of Chicago Press, 1993.
McCutcheon, Russell. *Critics Not Caretakers: Redescribing the Public Study of Religion.* Albany: State University of New York Press, 2001.
———. *Manufacturing Religion.* New York: Oxford University Press, 1997.
Neville, Robert Cummings. "Religious Studies and Theological Studies." *Journal of the American Academy of Religion* 61, no. 2: 185-200.
Ong, Walter J. *Orality and Literacy: The Technologizing of the Word.* London & New York: Routledge, 1982.
Otto, Rudolf. *The Idea of the Holy.* Tr. James Harvey. London & New York: Oxford University Press, 1958.

Penner, Hans H. *Impasse and Resolution: A Critique of the Study of Religion*. New York: Peter Lang, 1989.

Preus, J. Samuel. *Explaining Religion: Criticism and Theory from Bodin to Freud*. New Haven: Yale University Press, 1987.

Roberts, Tyler. "Exposure and Explanation: On the New Protectionism in the Study of Religion." *Journal of the American Academy of Religion*. 72, no. 1 (March 2004): 143-172.

Ryba, Thomas. *The Essence of Phenomenology and Its Meaning for the Scientific Study of Religions*. Vol. 7. New York: Peter Lang, 1991.

Said, Edward. *Orientalism*. New York: Pantheon Books, 1978.

Schechner, Richard. *Between Theater and Anthropology*. Philadelphia: University of Pennsylvania, 1985.

Schechner, Richard, and Willa Appel, eds. *By Means of Performance*. Cambridge, UK: Cambridge University Press, 1990.

Sharpe, Eric. *Comparative Religion: A History*. LaSalle, IL: Open Court, 1986.

Smith, Jonathan Z. *To Take Place: Toward Theory in Ritual*. Chicago: University of Chicago Press, 1987.

———. *Imagining Religion: From Jonestown to Babylon*. Chicago: University of Chicago Press, 1982.

Smith, Wilfred Cantwell. *The Meaning and End of Religion*. Minneapolis: Fortress Press, 1991 [1962].

Straus, Edwin. *Phenomenal Psychology*. New York: Basic Books, 1966.

Suleiman, Susan Rubin. *The Female Body in Western Culture*. Cambridge, MA: Harvard University Press, 1985.

Sullivan, Lawrence. "'Seeking an End to the Primary Text' or 'Putting an End to the Text as Primary.'"41-59 in *Beyond the Classics? Essays in Religious Studies and Liberal Education*. Eds. F.E. Reynolds and S.L. Burkhalter. Atlanta, GA: Scholars Press, 1990.

Suydam, Mary A, and Joanna E. Ziegler, eds. *Performance and Transformation: New Approaches to Late Medieval Spirituality*. New York: St. Martin's Press, 1999.

Taussig, Michael. *Mimesis and Alterity: A Particular History of the Senses*. New York: Routledge, 1993.

Taylor, Mark C., ed. *Critical Terms for Religious Studies*. Chicago: University of Chicago Press, 1998.

Torgovnick, Marianna. *Gone Primitive: Savage Intellects, Modern Lives*. Chicago: University of Chicago Press, 1990.

Turner, Victor. *The Ritual Process: Structure and Anti-Structure*. New York: Aldine de Gruyter, 1995 [1966].

———. *Dramas, Fields, and Metaphors: Symbolic Action in Human Society*. Ithaca, NY: Cornell University Press, 1974.

Wasserstrom, Steven P. *Religion after Religion: Gershom Scholem, Mircea Eliade, and Henry Corbin at Eranos*. Princeton: Princeton University Press, 1999.

Wiebe, Donald. *The Politics of Religious Studies*. New York: Palgrave Press, 1999.

Dance Studies: History and Theory

Albright, Ann Cooper. *Choreographing Difference*. Hanover, NH: Wesleyan University Press, 1997.

Armitage, Merle, ed. *Martha Graham: The Early Years*. New York: de Capo Press, 1978 [1937].

Banes, Sallie. *Dancing Women: Female Bodies on Stage*. New York: Routledge, 1998.

———. *Terpsichore in Sneakers: Post-modern Dance*. Boston: Houghton Mifflin, 1980.

———. *Writing Dancing in the Age of Postmodernism*. Hanover, NH: Wesleyan University Press, 1994.

Blair, Fredrika. *Isadora: Portrait of the Artist as a Woman*. New York: McGraw Hill, 1986.

Burt, Ramsey. *Alien Bodies*. New York: Routledge, 1998.

Carter, Alexandra, ed. *The Routledge Dance Studies Reader*. New York: Routledge, 1998.

Copeland, Roger, and Marshal Cohen, eds. *What Is Dance? Readings in Theory and Criticism*. New York: Oxford, 1983.

Daly, Ann. *Done into Dance: Isadora Duncan in America*. Bloomington, IN: Indiana University Press, 1995.

de Mille, Agnes. *Martha: The Life and Work of Martha Graham*. New York: Random House, 1991.

Desmond, Jane. "Dancing Out the Difference: Cultural Imperialism and Ruth St. Denis's 'Radha' of 1906." *Signs* 17, no. 1 (Autumn 1991): 28-49.

———, ed. *Meaning in Motion*. Durham, NC: Duke University Press, 1997.

Dils, Ann, and Ann Cooper Albright, eds. *Moving History/Dancing Cultures*. Middletown: Wesleyan University Press, 2001.

Duncan, Isadora. *The Art of the Dance*. New York: Theater Arts Books, 1977 [1928].

———. *My Life*. New York: Boni and Liveright, 1927.

The Early Years: American Modern Dance 1900-1930s. A conference at SUNY College, April 9-12 1981. Videotaped proceedings at NYPL.

Foster, Susan Leigh, ed. *Corporealities: Dancing Knowledge, Culture and Power*. London: Routledge, 1996.

———. *Choregraphing History*. Bloomington, IN: Indiana University Press, 1995.

———. *Reading Dancing: Bodies and Subjects in Contemporary American Dance*. Berkeley, CA: University of California Press, 1986.

Fraleigh, Sondra Horton. *Dance and the Lived Body: A Descriptive Aesthetics*. Pittsburgh: University of Pittsburgh Press, 1987.

Fraleigh, Sondra Horton, and Penelope Hanskin, eds. *Researching Dance: Evolving Modes of Inquiry*. Pittsburgh: University of Pittsburgh Press, 1999.

Franko, Mark. *Dancing Modernism/Performing Politics*. Bloomington, IN: Indiana University Press, 1995.

Garafola, Lynn, ed. *Rethinking the Sylph*. Hanover, NH: University Press of New England, 1997.

Garaudy, Roger. *Danser Sa Vie*. Paris: Editions du Seuil, 1973.

Hanna, Judith Lynne. *Dance, Sex, and Gender: Signs of Identity, Dominance, Defiance, and Desire*. Chicago: University of Chicago Press, 1988.

————. "The Representation and Reality of Religion in Dance." *Journal of the American Academy of Religion*. 61, no. 2 (1988): 281-300.

————. *To Dance Is Human*. Chicago: University of Chicago Press, 1987 [1979].

Jowitt, Deborah. *Time and the Dancing Image*. Berkeley, CA: University of California Press, 1988.

Kealiinohomoku, Joann. "Dance Ethnology: Where Do We Go from Here?" *Dancing in the Millennium Conference*, July 20, 2000.

————. "An Anthropologist Looks at Ballet as a Form of Ethnic Dance." 533-549 in *What Is Dance?* Eds. Roger Copeland and Marshal Cohen. New York: Oxford University Press, 1983.

Kendall, Elizabeth. *Where She Danced: The Birth of American Art-Dance*. Berkeley, CA: University of California Press, 1979.

LaMothe, Kimerer L. *Nietzsche's Dancers: Isadora Duncan, Martha Graham, and the Reevaluation of Christian Values*. New York: Palgrave, 2005.

————."Passionate Madonna: The Christian Turn of Ruth St. Denis." *Journal of the American Academy of Religion* 66, no. 4: 747-769.

Lloyd, Margaret. *The Borzoi Book of Modern Dance*. New York: Dance Horizons, 1949.

Loewenthal, Lillian. "Isadora Duncan in the Netherlands." *Dance Chronicle* 3, no. 3: (1979-80): 227-253.

Magriel, Paul, ed. *Chronicles of the American Dance: From the Shakers to Martha Graham*. New York: de Capo Press, 1978 [1948].

Manning, Susan. *Ecstasy and the Demon: Feminism and Nationalism in the Dances of Mary Wigman*. Berkeley, CA: University of California, 1993.

Manor, Giora. *The Gospel According to Dance: Choreography and the Bible from Ballet to Modern*. New York: St. Martin's Press, 1980.

Mazo, Joseph. *Prime Movers: The Makers of Modern Dance in America*. New York: Morrow, 1977.

Nadel, Myron Howard, and Constance Gwen Nadel, eds. *The Dance Experience: Readings in Dance Appreciation*. New York: Praeger Publishers, 1970.

Ness, Sally. *Body, Movement and Culture: Kinesthetic and Visual Symbolism in a Philippine Community*. Philadelphia: University of Pennsylvania Press, 1992.

Novack, Cynthia. *Sharing the Dance: Contact Improvisation and American Culture*. Wisconsin: University of Wisconsin Press, 1990.

Rogers, Frederick R., ed. *Dance: A Basic Educational Technique*. New York: MacMillan, 1941.

Sheets-Johnstone, Maxine. *The Primacy of Movement*. Amsterdam, Philadelphia: John Benjamins Publishing, 1999.

———. *The Roots of Thinking*. Philadelphia: Temple University Press, 1990.

———. *Illuminating Dance: Philosophical Explorations*. Cranbury, NJ: Associated University Press, 1984.

———. *The Phenomenology of Dance*. Madison: University of Wisconsin Press, 1966.

———, ed. *Giving the Body Its Due*. Albany, New York: SUNY Press, 1992.

Shelton, Suzanne. *Divine Dancer: A Biography of Ruth St. Denis*. Garden City, NY: Doubleday and Company, 1981.

Siegel, Marcia. *The Shapes of Change: Images of American Dance*. Boston: Houghton Mifflin, 1979.

Sklar, Deirdre. "On Dance Ethnography." *Dance Research Journal* 23, no. 1:6-10.

Sorrell, Walter. *Dance in Its Time*. New York: Columbia University Press, 1981.

———, ed. *The Dance Has Many Faces*. New York: Columbia University Press, 1966.

Sparshott, Francis. *Off the Ground: First Steps to a Philosophical Consideration of the Dance*. Princeton: Princeton University Press, 1988.

St. Denis, Ruth. *Ruth St. Denis, An Unfinished Life*. New York: Harper & Brothers Publishers, 1939.

———. *Lotus Light*. Cambridge, MA: The Riverside Press. 1932.

Terry, Walter. "Ruth St. Denis, Seventy, Heads Church of the Divine Dance." *New York Times*, July 13, 1947.

———. *Frontiers of the Dance: The Life of Martha Graham*. New York: Crowell, 1975.

Youngerman, Suzanne. "Curt Sachs and His Heritage: A Critical Review of World History of the Dance with a Survey of Recent Studies that Perpetuate His Ideas." *Dance Research Journal* 6, no. 2:6-19.

Christianity and Dance: History and Theology

Adams, Doug. *Congregational Dancing in Christian Worship*. Austin: The Sharing Company, 1971.

Adams, Doug, and Diane Apostolos-Cappadona, eds. *Dance as Religious Studies*. New York: Crossroad, 1990.

Ahlstrom, Sydney. *A Religious History of the American People.* New Haven: Yale, 1972.

———. *The People Called Shakers.* New York: Oxford University Press, 1953.

Andrews, Edward. *A Gift to Be Simple: Songs, Dances and Rituals of the American Shakers.* New York: J.J. Augustin Publisher, 1940.

Backman, Louis. *Religious Dances in the Christian Church and in Popular Medicine.* Tr. [from Swedish by] E. Classen. London: George Allen & Unwin Ltd., 1952.

Brown, Peter. *Body and Society: Men, Women, and Sexual Renunciation in Early Christianity.* New York: Columbia University Press, 1988.

Bynum, Carolyn Walker. *The Resurrection of the Body in Western Christianity, 200-1336.* New York: Columbia University Press, 1995.

Davies, J.G. *Liturgical Dance: An Historical, Theological, and Practical Handbook.* London: SCM Press, 1984.

———. "Towards a Theology of the Dance. 43-63 in *Worship and Dance.* Ed. J.G. Davies. University of Birmingham, ISWRA, 1975.

Fisk, Margaret Palmer. *The Art of the Rhythmic Choir.* New York: Harper and Brothers Publishers, 1950.

Gagne, Ronald, Thomas Kane, and Robert VerEecke. *Introducing Dance in Christian Worship.* Portland, OR: Pastoral Press, 1999.

Intravaia, Toni. *And We Have Danced.* Vol. 2. Henry Printing Inc., 1994.

Kraemer, Ross Shepard. *Her Share of the Blessings: Women's Religions among Pagans, Jews, and Christians in the Greco-Roman World.* New York: Oxford University Press, 1992.

Lawler, L.B. *The Dance in Ancient Greece.* Middletown, CT: Wesleyan University Press, 1978.

Miles, Margaret R. *Carnal Knowing: Female Nakedness and Religious Meaning in the Christian West.* New York: Vintage Books, Random House, 1991.

———. *Image as Insight: Visual Understanding in Western Christianity and Secular Culture.* Boston: Beacon Press, 1985.

———. *Fullness of Life: Historical Foundations for a New Asceticism.* Philadelphia: The Westminster Press, 1981.

Oesterley, W.O.E. *The Sacred Dance.* New York: Cambridge University Press, 1923.

Porterfield, Amanda. *Feminine Spirituality in America: From Sarah Edwards to Martha Graham.* Philadelphia: Temple University Press, 1980.

Raboteau, Albert. *Slave Religion.* Oxford University Press, 1978.

Reed, Carlynn. *And We Have Danced: A History of the Sacred Dance Guild, 1958-1978.* Austin, TX: The Sharing Co., 1978.

Rock, Judith. *Theology in the Shape of Dance.* Austin, TX: The Sharing Company, 1978.

Rock, Judith, and Norman Mealy. *Performer as Priest and Prophet: Restoring the Intuitive in Worship through Music and Dance.* New York: Harper and Row, 1988.

Sachs, Curt. *A World History of Dance.* Tr. Bessie Schonberg. New York: W.W. Norton, 1937.

Sacred Dance Guild Journal 37, no. 2 (Winter 1995).

A Summary View of the Millennial Church or United Society of Believers (Commonly Called Shakers) Comprising the Rise, Progress and Practical Order of the Society, Together with the General Principles of Their Faith and Testimony. Albany: Packard and van Benthuysen, 1848 [1823].

Taylor, Margaret Fisk. *A Time to Dance: Symbolic Movement in Worship.* Austin, TX: The Sharing Co., 1981 [1967, 76, 78].

Wagner, Ann. *Adversaries of Dance: From the Puritans to the Present.* Urbana, IL: University of Illinois Press, 1997.

Gerardus van der Leeuw

Carman, John. "The Theology of a Phenomenologist: An Introduction to the Theology of Gerardus van der Leeuw." *Harvard Divinity School Bulletin* 29, no. 3 (April 1965): 13-42.

Hermelink, Jan. *Verstehen und Bezeugen: Der theologische Ertrag der 'Phänomenologie der Religion' von Gerardus van der Leeuw.* Munchen: Chr. Kaiser Verlag, 1960.

Hubbeling, H.G. *Divine Presence in Ordinary Life: Gerardus van der Leeuw's Twofold Method in His Thinking on Art and Religion.* Amsterdam: North Holland Publishing Company, 1986.

Kippenberg, Hans G., and Brigitte Luchesi, eds. *Religionswissenschaft und Kulturkritik: Beitrage zur Konfrenz—The History of Religions and Critique of Culture in the Days of Gerardus van der Leeeuw (1890-1950).* Marburg: diagonal-Verlag, 1991.

van der Leeuw, Gerardus. "Confession Scientifique: Faites à l'Université Masaryk de Bruno, Le lundi 18 novembre 1946." *Numen: International Review for the History of Religions.* Volume I. Leiden: E.J. Brill, 1954, 8-15.

——. *Godsvoorstellingen in de oud-Ægyptische pyramideteksten.* Th. D. dissertation, University of Leiden, 1916.

——. *"In dem Himmel ist ein Tanz . . ." Über die religiöse Bedeutung des Tanzes und des Festzuges.* Munchen, 1931.

——. *In den hemel is enen dance.* Amsterdam, 1930.

——. *Inleiding tot de godsdienstgeschiedenis.* Haarlem, 1924. De erven F. Bohn, 1948.

——. *Inleiding tot de theologie.* Second edition. Amsterdam: H.J. Paris, 1948.

————. *Phänomenologie der Religion.* Tübingen: Verlag von J.C.B. Mohr, 1933.

————. *La religion dans son essence et ses manifestations. Phénoménologie de la religion,* Paris: Payot, 1948. [1955, 1970]

————. *Religion in Essence and Manifestation.* Tr. J.E. Turner. Princeton: Princeton University Press, 1986.

————. *Sacramentstheologie.* Nijkerk: G. F. Callenback, 1949.

————. *Sacred and Profane Beauty: The Holy in Art.* Tr. David E. Green. New York: Holt, Rhinehart, & Winston, 1963.

————. *Vom Heiligen und der Kunst.* Tr. Frau Dr. A. Piper. Carl Bertelsmann Verlag: Gutersloh, 1957.

————. *Wegen en grenzen. Studie over de verhouding van religie en kunst.* Second edition. Amsterdam: H. J. Paris, 1948.

————. *Wegen en Grenzen. Studie over de verhouding van religie en kunst.* Third edition prepared by E.S. Smelik. Amsterdam: H. J. Paris, 1955.

Waardenburg, Jacques. "Religion between Reality and Idea: A Century of Phenomenology of Religion in the Netherlands." *Numen* 19 (1971): 128-203.

————. *Classical Approaches to the Study of Religion. Religion and Reason 3: Method and Theory in the Study and Interpretation of Religion.* The Hague: Mouton, 1973.

————. "Reflections on the Study of Religion, Including an Essay on the Work of Gerardus van der Leeuw." *Religion and Reason* 15. The Hague: Mouton Publishers, 1978.

Index

"Acts of John," 198–99
Art, 171; as sacred or profane, 174
Asad, Talal, 5

Bell, Catherine, 5–6
Bodily becoming, logic of, 183: and culture, 188; as enacting what it means to be "human," 225
Body: and dance, 181–84; as an object for religious studies, 246–47; in modern consciousness, 220. *See also* Physical consciousness

Culture: and dance, 184–88; as spiral of discovery and response, 185–88, 195–96

Dance, 2; and eroticism, 217–18; and theater, 216–17; and writing, 235; ballet, 91–93; in Christianity, 2, 9–10, 197, 198–99, 216–18, 257, 259n1; learning to, 234–35; object for religious studies, 229–31; of couples, 190; paradigm for other arts, 200–205; religious dance, 212–13; resource for theory and method in religious studies, 243–55. *See also* Hovering dances; Striding dances

Descartes, René: God, 27–28; on experience, 25–28; on religion, 28–29; use of reason, 25–28
Disconcerting miracle, 231
Drama, 204
Duncan, Isadora, 8–9, 160

Ecstatic dances. *See* Hovering dances
Eliade, Mircea, 174
Emergence narrative, 3–6, 10–12; critique of, 19–20, 103–5
Enlightenment, 7, 21–25; and religion, 52–53; criticism of knowledge paradigms, 244
Epoche, 147–49. *See also* Phenomenological method
Essence, 140–42; of a phenomenon, 131–32, 134, 140–42
Experience: as resource for religious studies, 22–25, 233–34; imaginative recreation of, 143–47

Foucault, Michel, 5, 162, 238, 263n1, 276n5

Hegel, G. W. F.: and dance, 84; and religious studies, 73–74; and writing, 80–83; critique of earlier theories of religion, 65–68, 71–72; on religion, 70–73; on Science,

on, 119–22. *See also* Hegel; Kant; Kierkegaard; Religion; Schleiermacher; Writing

Understanding: as full-bodied action, 233; as love, 239; practice of, 143–52. *See also* Imaginative empathy; Phenomenological method
Unity of life, 179

Van der Leeuw, Gerardus, 109–13, 126–28; attitudes towards dance, 159–60; defining art, 171; defining

religion, 161–66; on experience, 139–40; translation of, 110, 173–75, 275n4, 277n16; value of, 11, 235–40. *See also* Phenomenological method; Phenomenology of religion

Weber, Max, 134
Writing: about dance, 206–9; as bodily practice, 207, 234–35, 254–56, 105–6; in relation to theology, 219; in the study of religion, 4–5, 7, 168–70, 254–56